GW00870343

1

TOO SEXY FOR ALS:

How to fight for your life with everything you got!

by
Elizabeth Ann Smith

Published by Elizabeth Ann Smith
ISBN 978-0-359-28511-2

Too

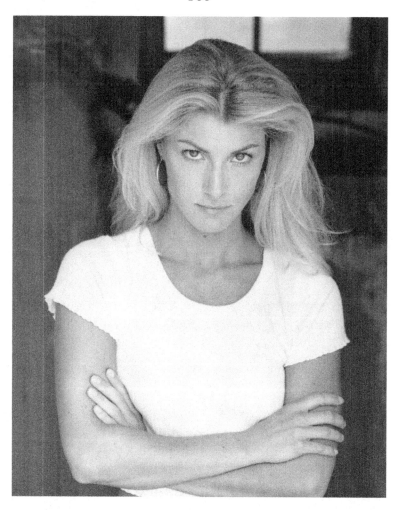

Sexy

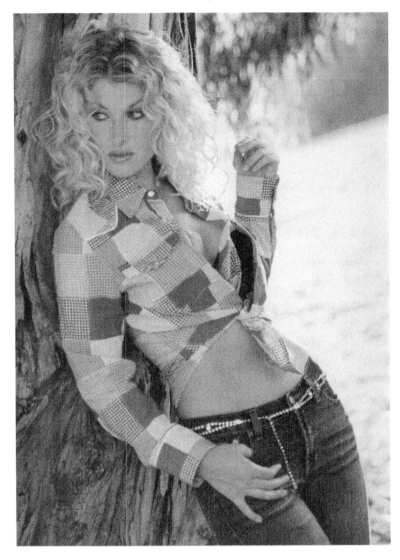

For

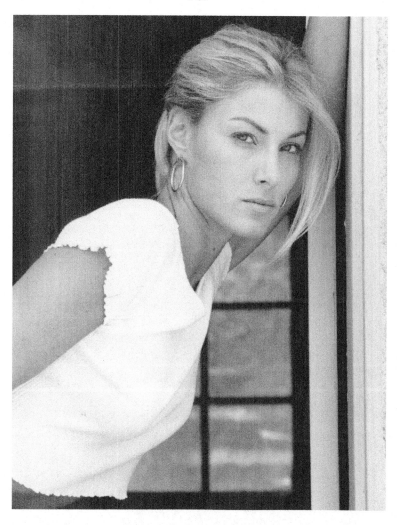

ALS

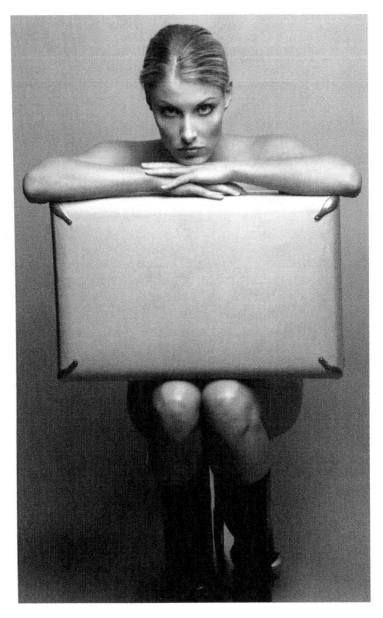

Dedication

I would like to dedicate this book to every caregiver who helped me get out of bed where I was for three years. Your hard work and dedication has made this one of my best years thus far. Since my first short trip out of bed in June of 2017, we have accomplished a great deal and I am grateful to you for each part you have played. You are my badass hos: Jenny Askeland, Amanda Adair, Mandi Dillmann, and Carie Ericsson. I would also like to thank Alena Martinez for your attentiveness at night that surely helps me get more sleep than I would get otherwise. Lastly, I would like to thank my dad for supporting me and my caregivers. Your presence makes a difference! Love you dad.

This book is brought to life on audio book by Serene Zloof available at www.toosexyformybedpan.org

Too Sexy For ALS: How to fight for your life with everything you got!

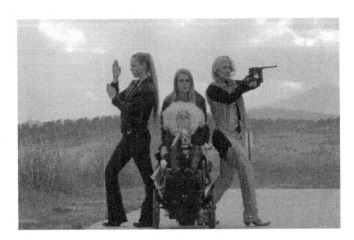

Table of Contents

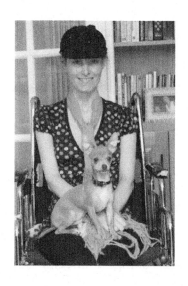

ABOUT THE AUTHOR

Elizabeth Ann Smith was born and raised near Kansas City, Missouri. Elizabeth is a graduate of Florida Atlantic University and the University of Missouri, Kansas City. An avid traveler, she has a love of diverse cultures. As a member of the Screen Actors' Guild, she acted in several movies, made TV appearances, was a comic book character and performed stand-up comedy in Los Angeles, California. She worked for a private law firm, pharmaceutical companies, was a bilingual spokesperson for luxury car manufacturers while also selling their cars, and owned her own textile business called, Christian Chicks, LLC. In 2005 at the age of 30,

Elizabeth began experiencing symptoms of ALS or Lou Gehrig's disease while training for a marathon. She resides and manages her team of caregivers in northern Colorado.

Elizabeth is currently writing a series of books to help both caregivers and those receiving care. All are available on her website, toosexyformybedpan.org. She writes her books using a special computer and by blinking her eyes to select each letter. Her first book, *Too Sexy for My Bedpan: How to Give and Receive Care* was published in late 2017 and gives her personal story. Her second and third books, *Too Sexy for ALS: How to Fight for Your Life with Everything You Got!* and *Too Sexy for My Caregiver: How to Find and Manage Good Care*, are set to be published in late 2018 and early 2019. After being cared for by nearly 400 caregivers, Elizabeth has learned a bit about what works! Faith and humor are her keys to success.

Follow her at
www.facebook.com/toosexyformybedpan/

YouTube channel, Too Sexy for My Bedpan:

https://www.youtube.com/channel/UCQFW5JB070lhn UelhmyTY8Q

Too Sexy for My Bedpan trailer:
https://www.youtube.com/watch?v=1vcl4OiVhOo

Babeforce trailer:
https://www.youtube.com/watch?v=dc1TiV9dVaY

Who Wants to Be a Princess? (the entire show):
https://vimeo.com/243374401/593d7a09e4

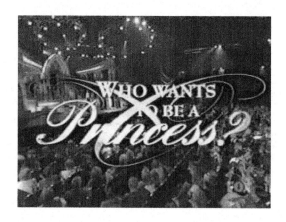

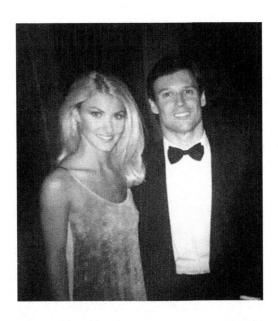

Elizabeth with the Prince of Rome, Guglielmo Giovanelli Marconi at MGM Grand Hotel, Las Vegas, after the filming of the Fox television show, "Who Wants to be a Princess," before a live audience of over two thousand people. She was also privileged to meet his mother, Marchesa Maria Elettra Elena Anna Marconi (daughter of the man who invented the radio).

FORWARD

This book is NOT about ALS. I could care less about ALS, cancer, MS, or any other ugly disease that rears its head. I do not give disease the time of day. All disease can kiss my ever living, never-seen-the-sun butt! I have often thought that instead of giving a whole month to things like Breast Cancer Awareness (sponsored by dairy companies when there is a direct link to breast cancer and dairy!), this nation should be making people aware of ways to stay healthy or ways to be healed. Through educating people about our corrupt food supply or the fact that Jesus Christ heals, we could prevent many diseases by changing people's diet and give hope to those receiving a diagnosis. Of course, that becomes political, and would put most food industries completely out of business. People would get offended by the mixing of religion with government, but let's not forget that we are a Christian nation from inception. Not to reduce the physical trials people are going through, but wouldn't it behoove the public to be more aware of how to get healthy than merely being aware of all these diseases? Some examples I can think of: Organic

Awareness, National Lay Hands on Somebody Day (get your mind out of the gutter!), What's in Your Meat Month, National Eat Dirt Day, Fermentation Awareness Month, and Let the Lame Walk Month. What are we really gaining by becoming more aware of disease? Disease awareness is nothing but a fear campaign that empowers disease in our consciousness!

I have never identified with disease. I have not been to one ALS Association meeting. I have never attended an ALS Clinic where many specialists visit patients. And I have never participated in a walk for ALS. If it helps you to do that sort of thing, go for it! ALS is just a diagnosis. I am too busy living to think about ALS. If you want to have a Strong and Fearless rally, I'm all in! You become who you surround yourself with. If you surround yourself with people who think and talk disease and symptoms, that is what you're going to get. The two people I knew who had ALS died and they never missed a meeting. I don't find that particularly encouraging. Can you imagine going to ALS Association meetings for as long as I have been fighting ALS? Think about all of the people who have died in thirteen years! I'm sorry, count me out. I want to survive and must keep my eyes on the prize. That may seem selfish to you, but my contribution are my books, and I believe they are helping people think differently.

I am not involved with the ALS Association. When I was first diagnosed, my doctor arranged for me to meet with them. If I remember correctly, they talked to me and my husband about the social service part of things, like setting up an advance directive, a will and a DNR (and burial!). I mean, what the hell? No wonder people die so quickly! Don't they realize what that can do to someone who is not strong? If I was not strong, I can imagine wanting to blow my brains out after meeting with them! No wonder people don't believe they can beat this. In Oregon, they talked to my husband about putting me in a home right in front of me as if I was a crazy person just because of my diagnosis! In Colorado, they wouldn't allow my caregiver to talk about my book or hand out flyers, something that could actually help someone. I have seen their advertisements and they bring in speakers that tell you how to get your affairs in order or physicians who tell you what you can expect as far as the progression goes. Who needs that? Nobody has the right to tell me or you what will happen to our bodies. I am curious to know how much of their fundraising actually goes to research. They are a huge organization and have a lot of overhead. I'm sure they help people (yeah, get to their grave!), but don't forget that disease is big business. I was wondering what they do to help people, so I went on their website. I was shocked and appalled to see a picture of the doctor who diagnosed me! He is on their payroll! When he diagnosed me, he said rotten things that you should never say to anyone facing that type of a diagnosis. In fact, one of the things he said to me was not only untrue, but I won't even repeat it as long as I live- it was so terrible. I am fed up at this point. If you want to donate to organizations that pay doctors big bucks, that is your business, but it disgusts me. I can only speak from my personal experience with them and I would like to see them play a role in encouraging people to fight this disease instead of accepting it. I don't believe they are remotely interested in a cure. They would have to find another cause to leach from!

I have recently become friends with people who have ALS on Facebook and I enjoy reading about the people who are out living and not talking about disease.

Unfortunately, many of them allow their lives to be run by the disease and every post has the word ALS in it. Your diagnosis doesn't have to be your life. There is one gentleman who messaged me and said that he doesn't live with the disease and makes the disease live with him! He is one of the few people I have found who is not catering to the disease and he was diagnosed 19 years ago! My heart goes out to these people. I love them all and know all too well the pain they're going through. I have been asked to go to DC to tell my story and to write my congressmen. I thought about it and realized that if I did, I would be claiming the disease-when the Bible says I am healed. I am not about to sign for THAT package! If the disease is your identity or becomes your purpose in life, you will never beat it.

My principle motivation for writing this book is to give people hope. You were given a terminal diagnosis, so what? Everyone's terminal. Millions of people are given a terminal diagnosis each year. Your response to the diagnosis is what can make you unique. It's time to hunker down and fight. Are you really going to let this pathetic disgusting disease take your life? Life is worth fighting for no matter who you are or what you have in life. This is your opportunity to do something meaningful with your life. If you have ever felt that your life has never made much of an impact, here's your chance. Maybe you don't know that you have authority over disease. What if you die? What if you don't? It's much better to live in bravery than fear.

I am not a physician and don't have all the answers, but I do have thirteen years of experience overcoming a deadly disease. If only I knew then what I know now! I have become very bold. Our medical system will kill you if you give them a chance! There's a reason why they call it a medical PRACTICE. According to Francis Raymond in his book, *Never Be Sick Again*, over one million deaths each year are caused by modern medicine-which is the leading cause of death in our country. I attribute my success to strong faith, positive attitude, high quality nutrition, humor, good caregivers who are unsympathetic, not caring what people think and staying in learning mode. You will never regret fighting for your life.

CHAPTER ONE

THE WILL TO LIVE

I f you don't have the will to live, this is the first thing you must change. For a long time I struggled with my reasons for wanting to live. I always have had a very strong desire to live as most people do, but I couldn't seem to come up with reasons that seemed worthy. I don't have a husband anymore or children (which might be a good thing now that I think about it!). I don't really have a career, per say. I manage my team, but sometimes that is enough to drive you crazy. If you have ever managed people, you know that it can be next to impossible to keep everyone happy. I sort of felt condemned by not having a good reason for living. Religious programs talk about having a purpose and a destiny. Even Tony Robbins, who I get a lot from, talks about the WHY being an important factor in your action plan. While I feel that I do have a purpose and destiny that includes bringing hope to others as well as the awesome news of the gospel and freedom in Christ; that is not my motivation for living.

Find your Reasons

I want to live because it's fun! I believe I will not always be in this physical condition. Faith has empowered me and God has given me all the tools I need to be his copilot in creating health and full recovery in my body. I am only in my early forties and would like to have a family and become a chef. I would like to take care of my parents when and if they need it. I want to do many things that constitute living and I know the Lord wants that for me too. If you have been given a terminal diagnosis, have the courage to step out and believe that this too shall pass in this lifetime. You must participate in your recovery with works of faith. One of the most important things you have to change is the words coming out of your mouth. Nothing good can happen if you continue to talk about what the doctors say. For a long time I didn't have the faith to speak positive, but I knew enough to not speak against myself. Speech is a very powerful gift we have been given. We get what we say. We have to learn to say the things we want and not what we have! One person who has mastered this is President Trump. If you listen to what he is saying, everything is the greatest and the best. He is constantly prophesying over his own life and look at where he is now! He speaks his faith and it comes to pass! He doesn't care if people think he's an idiot and many people do. You can not value the opinion of man over God. I could care less what people think about me believing that I have already been healed. They are the fools!

It was not until recently that I discovered some of the other reasons I truly want to live. I guess you could say that all of my reasons fall under the joy of living. One of the greatest joys of this life for me is making someone laugh. It is often strangers or anyone really. It's not that I think I am that funny or anything. I just enjoy saying things that people don't expect and making them smile and gasp with laughter. I guess this is why I tried out stand-up comedy in Hollywood. My act was about growing up with a brother who was often in jail. I joked about visiting him on holidays and going to the park with him to sell 'pre-owned' merchandise like hubcaps, instead of doing normal brother and sister stuff. Immediately following my surgery to install the tracheostomy, I met with my pulmonologist to discuss how it was going to change my life. When he walked into my room I said, "Does this trach make me look fat?" He was drinking coffee and he literally choked and had to spit it out. That is fun. Recently I had an x-ray taken of my throat and head. As the handsome ENT was showing me the results, I was appalled at the image and said, "OMG! I look wretched! Take that down!" He about died. I had a new caregiver who had Sunday off and went to church. During the service I texted her, 'May the Lord be a light unto your path to find my butthole.' That is fun. We were at a concert and went to the lobby for intermission. This lady came over to pet Nutter Butter and started talking about chihuahuas. She asked me if hip dysplasia was common in chihuahuas as if I was a vet. I replied, "All I know is that they have extremely large penises." She screamed with laughter and awkwardly departed. That is fun. I am sure it is a bit prideful thinking that I am bringing people joy, but I have a good time!

One of my other reasons for living is to enjoy beauty. One day I was listening to a station of orchestral music. This music was so incredibly beautiful it brought tears to my eyes. I was thanking God that I was alive just to hear that song. When I look out the window, the beauty overwhelms me. The leaves hang on the trees like crystals from a chandelier. Rich or poor, I have always surrounded myself with beauty. My home doesn't look like the home of someone who the world calls disabled. I have never equipped my homes with a bunch of medical crap. First of all, it is ugly. And who wants to be reminded of your situation? When I used to be transferred to my recliner, I would have my caregiver put the wheelchair in the other room so I didn't have to look at it. People need to be reminded of the possibilities, not of their current situation. I store my hoyer, shower chair and any other ugly medical junk in the garage, that is until I can blow it up with dynamite! Have you ever seen a shower chair? OMG! It looks like an electric chair! Trust me, you will wish it were if you stare at it long enough!

I would like to talk about a friend of mine who died. He was diagnosed with ALS around the same time I was 13 years ago. We met after I moved to Colorado. I knew him five years. We both lived in our own homes and managed our care team. When I went on Facebook and saw all of the tributes to him, I was shocked. Was it a freak accident? He had never given me any indication that he was ready to give up. I couldn't believe he died because he had just called me 'Barbie' on one of my pictures on Facebook. I asked around and apparently he refused treatment at a local hospital. This didn't sound like him and I was baffled. I met with his family two months later and learned the very sad story of what really happened. He was having trouble getting out of bed and was faced with the two options of either being bedbound or using a hoyer (like I do). He was not open to either one and had a family member call hospice. He had given up. A week after he expressed his will to die, a bizarre infection came upon him and he started having seizures due to low sodium. The devil is more than happy to accommodate your wishes if you want to die. "The thief cometh not, but for to steal, and to kill and to destroy; I am come that they may have life and that they might have it more abundantly." (John 10:10 KJV) I knew there was more to the story of his death! It gave me chills. Why didn't he talk to me about using a hoyer? It is not difficult once you practice. I can't judge him, and I don't know what he was going through. It just seemed totally unnecessary to me. What happened to my friend shows how critical the will to live really is. The bible says that it is our choice to lay down our life (John 10:18).

Find your Goals

This is what Wikipedia has to say about the will to live: "There are significant correlations between the will to live and existential, psychological, social, and physical sources of distress. The concept of the will to live can be seen as directly impacted by hope. Many, who overcome near-death experiences with no explanation, have described the will to live as a direct component of their survival. The difference between the wish to die versus the wish to live is also a unique risk factor for suicide."[1]

Hope, as defined by Wikipedia, "is a state of mind that is based on an expectation of positive outcomes with respect to events and circumstances in one's life or the world at large. As a verb, its definitions include: 'expect with confidence' and 'to cherish a desire with anticipation.'"[2]

I expect with confidence that I will leave sickness behind and soon. I cherish many desires with

---

[1] https://en.wikipedia.org/wiki/Will_to_live
[2] https://en.wikipedia.org/wiki/Hope

anticipation, including: eating several plates full of crispy shredded hash browns smothered in ketchup, tweezing my eyebrows, cooking for my friends and family and healing the sick though the power of God. I also look forward to the things I have planned in the short term like concerts, shopping, decorating for each holiday, and trips to Denver.

I have always been full of hope. Life is a kick in the pants so you might as well have some fun. I don't expect life to be a kick in the pants, but when it is, let the games begin! I grew up with a stressed out single mother who was always yelling. At a very young age my brother and I would be getting yelled at and we would laugh at my mother. Not out of disrespect, but the things she would say was hilarious. Three of my favorite things that she would say are: "eat your meat!" "Hell's bells!" and "shit damn!" It still makes me laugh today when I remember those times. It was certainly great training for life to find something to laugh about in the midst of trouble.

I am not just trying to hang on for medical research to come up with a cure. I'm not stupid and would surely take it if I still needed it, but I have little faith in anything medical. My hope and trust is in God and I enjoy the severe independence from people that my faith in God provides. I still need people in my life, but it has set me free from their opinions.

In order to have hope, it's necessary to have some goals. Your goals don't need to be laborious. One of my goals is to go to every museum in Denver. I enjoy planning the trips as much as I enjoy going. First off, I find the museum's free entrance days because paying for tickets for my entourage gets expensive. I search YouTube for videos on the museum and learn about its significance to the community, the design and architecture of the building, or its history. I even do this for places I'm not going to yet, like MOMA in New York City. This stimulates my mind and boosts my creativity. If you have always wanted to go somewhere, start learning about it as if you're going next month! It's exciting and will give you something else to focus on besides the dismal situation that surrounds you. Dream about being there. It is wonderful for your soul. I have not always been a Pollyanna. I have had to learn to find ways to enrich my soul and its importance.

Learn

Learn something new and it will foster your will to live. You are not truly living if you are not growing. Whatever you need to work on in your life or whatever interests you, decide to be a learner. If you need to work on your emotional life like I do, seek out books or videos that will help you. If your marriage sucks, learn what you can do to turn it around. I became a vegan and listened to several books on the microbiome and fitness. I love audiobooks because I use my eyes to type all day long and they allow them to rest. These books taught me so much and I created a new diet based on what I learned. The fitness book was about fighting middle age and was very motivating.

Create

We were made in God's image and he is the original creator. Nothing makes you feel more alive than when you are creating. It's one of the most pleasurable things humans experience. Entrepreneurship is creation. The arts are creation. Cooking is creation. If all you can make is a mess, go for it! Creation gives you a reason to live.

Music and movement

Get out of your funk. Music is a wonderful way to transport you to a different place. In the winter when there is snow covering the ground, I turn on Hawaiian music and pretend I am by the pool at a plush resort drinking a pina colada. The best investment I have ever made is in an Amazon Echo. I use it every day, all day. Anything I can imagine, she will play. It helps change the mood and infuse energy into the environment. If you aren't able to get an Echo, Pandora is a wonderful app for your computer or phone. When I poop, we play Roses, by Outcast. When I do my hair in pom poms, we play Big Balls, by ACDC. When we train someone on suctioning, we play Dirty Deeds, also by ACDC. When I ask my caregivers to do something that they would rather not, I play Whistle While You Work. I must be getting old because I am listening to classical music more often. I love listening to opera like Andrea Bocelli and pretend I am on the balcony of my Italian villa being serenaded by my lover, Giuseppe. My white scarf is hanging on to my neck as the wind carries the fresh scent of basil from the trattoria below. Giuseppe can no longer control his passion and plants a big kiss on me!

His muscles envelop my body! OMG! This is exactly how I dreamed it would happen! Okay, we had better stop there, but this is what music can do for you if you use it right. Exercise and music are a great combination to get you out of your funk. Move anything you can and keep moving it. Stop saying you can't! If you don't feel good, this will make you feel better. Try to get your heart pumping. The blood flowing through your body will completely change your state of mind, which is exactly what you need. In this altered state, you think differently. Creative ideas will come to you.

Be Competitive

Being competitive can help with having a fierce will to live. I could not stand losing at tennis. In college, I learned to play the sport. I lived in a condominium with all retired people. I would try to solicit singles games with old ladies. One of them had a pacemaker. Little did they know I was out for blood. One lady brought brownies to the court because I guess she assumed this was going to be a social thing. She was still trying to talk to me when I nailed a serve that was not returnable. That shut her up real quick. It probably sounds horrible, but I was there to play tennis just like I'm here right now with the purpose of fulfilling my destiny. The Hell am I going to let some sickness win this game. Even if I didn't really want to live, I think I would keep living just to keep the sickness from winning. I recently learned that I got my competitiveness from my dad. At our Fourth of July party, he put everyone to shame with the ho race. The goal was to pump the manual hoyer (hence why I call my girls 'hos'!) lift from its lowest position to its highest position in the least amount of time. You can tell that he never considered letting anyone else win. He did something no one else did and got on one knee to give himself more leverage. By the look on his face while he was pumping, you could see that he was determined to win at any cost. He smoked everyone. Nobody even came close to his time. At 75 years old, that is not too shabby! Here is a picture of us that day. We are wearing our team shirts that read, "Small hands, BIG balls! Go Trump!"

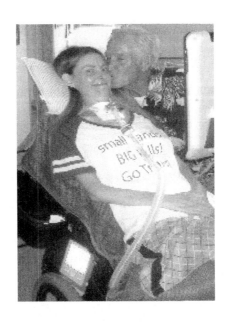

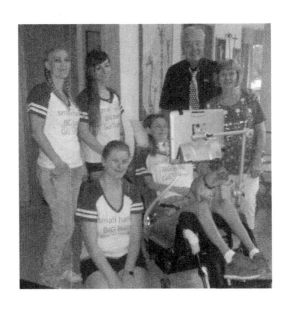

CHAPTER TWO

WEAPONS

Authority

Every one of us has authority over sickness and disease. Make disease your slave instead of the other way around. Didn't know you could? Absolutely! "Behold, I give unto you power to tread on serpents and scorpions and over all of the power of the enemy: and nothing by any means shall harm you." (Luke 10:19) "And God said, let us make man in our image, after our likeness: and let them have dominion over the fish of the sea, the fowl of the air, the cattle, all the earth and over every living thing that lives on the earth." (Genesis 1:26) We have dominion over disease because it is living. Tell disease to 'Scram!' Tell symptoms to go. For more on this topic, please listen to the best teaching I have found on this or search YouTube for "The believer's authority" by Andrew Wommack.[3]

---

[3] "The believer's authority" by Andrew Wommack: https://www.youtube.com/watch?v=E8K2hESIO-w&list=PLMSOSsad0PXIw0wEaDD_Y7r6emCMmntvG

Your thoughts

"As a man thinketh in his heart, so is he." (Proverbs 23:7) If you think you're weak, you are. If you think you're strong, you are. I once fired a lady because she was always saying, "I can't". As far as I am concerned, those are two words nobody should ever allow to come out of their mouth because they are self-defeating. If I am depending on you for my life, you better say, I will get this! Henry Ford once said, "Whether you think you can or you can't, your right." Your life is directed by your thoughts. Your thoughts have led you to where you are in life at this moment. You cannot let your mind wander on negative things. When you have a negative thought, cast it out. Change the channel. Thoughts are seeds from which all action originates. James Allen puts it this way in his book, *As a Man Thinketh*: "action is the blossom of thought and joy and suffering are its fruits. Thus does a man garner in the sweet and bitter fruitage of his own husbandry." Nothing good can come from bad thoughts. Only good can come from good thoughts. I learned this late in the game. It's a constant effort. Your will to live is determined by what you allow yourself to think about. You are in control of what you think about! Don't allow yourself to think about what you can no longer do or all that you have lost. Focus on the things you can do and all the things you have. "Finally, brethren, whatsoever things are true, whatsoever things are honest, whatsoever things are just, whatsoever things are pure, whatsoever things are lovely, whatsoever things are of good report, if there be any virtue, and if there be any praise, think on these things." (Philippians 4:8)

Recently, I had a revelation. I was listening to the song Le Vie En Rose.[4] I don't know French and was wondering what the lyrics meant. I looked it up and they are so sweet! Then I looked up the English translation for the title and it means 'life in pink' or 'looking at life with rose colored glasses'. I love this! This is how we should live! I just love that saying. I never used to like the color pink. I resented everything it stood for and it was way too girly for me. Since I became a Christian, so much has changed. I have learned the value of peace, honor and love. Heck, I

---

[4] Here's a beautiful video in English, enjoy!
https://www.youtube.com/watch?v=dqRq6qF7YgY

didn't know what love was! Pink now represents my new life (in Christ). Every time I think the words "pink life," my spirit soars. It's who I am. Enjoy the beautiful video in the footnote!

Your words

I am a huge word person. Most people don't pay attention to their words and just ramble on aimlessly. They do not realize that they are paving the way for their future and that they are where they are where they are right now because of their words. This is the only advantage of not being able to speak. As I have to type everything I say, I can really think about whether it is something I want to put out in the universe for myself. I have the opportunity to change what I am saying. If you had to write down everything you said, you would say much less and choose your words more carefully merely because of the amount of work involved. I come from a family of talkers and I tend to be one too. We sit around and talk. We talk about the weather and who died and catch up on what all of our mutual acquaintances are doing. We also have a tendency to talk about any ailment or sickness we have. This is where we say things like 'my arthritis' or 'my diabetes' and say things like I'm as blind as a bat or my back is killing me. This is dangerous territory. You will get everything you say. It is not just harmless chatter. "For assuredly, I say to you, whoever says to this mountain, 'be removed and be cast into the sea', and does not doubt in his heart, but believes those things that he says will be done, he will have whatever he says." (Mark 11:23) This is a powerful verse, but it can work for you or against you. How empowering that we can speak to our mountains and they will change if we believe. On the other hand, we say many things that are bad that we also believe and get what we say every single time. Do you say things like, 'I'm so clumsy; nothing good happens in my life; with my luck something bad will happen'? Sometimes we speak out of fear and cause the thing we fear the most to come to pass. One of my Facebook friends would always post about her daughter who had a rare disease. She would say that she was getting worse and bought everything the doctors told her. When I saw her posts, it broke my heart because she was cursing her unknowingly. Of course, she died. Yes, I am saying that your words can be the determining factor in whether you live or die. Instead of saying what was happening and that she was getting worse, she could have said what she wanted to have happen with faith. She could have declared, my daughter is strong and this disease will not take her life!

I have allowed myself to be cursed twice that I am aware of. I had a caregiver five years ago that was poisonous. She was always saying that what had happened to another ALS client she cared for was going to happen to me. This is exactly why I don't want caregivers who have cared for people with the diagnosis of ALS caring for me! The night she told me that I would definitely end up with a trach, I got so furious that I kicked her out of my house before I had the chance to get transferred to bed or use the restroom and slept in my recliner all night holding my pee! The bible says that we have been given an inheritance of condemning any words spoken against us (Isaiah 54:17). I didn't condemn her words and just got mad. Another time I believe I allowed myself to be cursed is when a respiratory therapist told me that my neck would atrophy. I just thought what an idiot he is, but I didn't condemn his words. A couple years later, a pediatric trach collar doesn't even fit me. Talking about what we have is natural and we all do it. Changing your speech to direct what you want and applying faith takes effort. "You will decree a thing and it will be established for you; and light will shine on your ways." (Job 22:28) Start establishing health in your body. "I will not die, but live and declare the works of the Lord." (Psalms 118:17) Use your speech to change your body even if you cannot speak with your mouth. If you have to just think it or use a device to speak, the important part is that you believe it. Tell your body how it's going to be from now on. Make the decision to be healthy. Once you make a decision, grace will follow. Speak to your mountain and to your body. I did this for two big toenails that were thick with fungus. I cursed fungus and commanded it to leave. I did this while my caregiver was putting my shoes on in the morning. I didn't even do it every morning! Within a year, both toenails were perfectly healed. The left one cleared first in about six months and then the right one started to change. That's all I did. I never used medication or anything. Isn't faith awesome? Writing this has gotten me all riled up. I am strong, healthy and whole. No disease or sickness will ever kill me! All disease that is in my body is leaving right now as I speak! I will only allow health in my body! My days of sickness and disease are over! "By Jesus' stripes, I was healed." (1 Peter 2:24). Everything changes when you understand that you have already been healed and are coming from a place of victory, but I will be covering this in a later chapter. I declare right now that many people will be healed as they read this book!

The word of God

The word of God is a weapon. Spoken and meditated on, it is the best way to ward off evil and disease. "My son, attend to my words; incline your ear to my words. Let them not depart from thine eyes; keep them in the midst of thine heart. For they are life to those that find them and medicine to all their flesh." (Proverbs 4:21-22) God's word is medicine for your flesh and you cannot overdose and there are zero side effects. It takes discipline to devote time to get into God's word every day and I am guilty of letting the cares of this life distract me. I'm the dummy because it is the best thing I could possibly do. Writing this book may just be the key to returning to the word every day because it's connecting the dots for me. Don't get me wrong, I play the Bible while I am sleeping most nights and I listen to great preachers all the time, but I am talking about focusing on healing scriptures each day. For a long, awesome list of healing scriptures, go to my website www.toosexyformybedpan.org. God's word is actually referred to as a sword, a fire and a hammer. "For the word of God is quick, and powerful, and sharper than any two-edged sword, piercing even to the dividing asunder of soul and spirit, and of the joints and marrow, and is a discerner of the thoughts and intents of the heart." (Hebrews 4:12) To someone who has been fighting disease more than a decade, the words 'quick' and 'powerful' are extremely appealing. Every time you speak healing scriptures over your body, you're stabbing the disease. How cool is that? "Is not my word like a fire, says the Lord, is it not like a mighty hammer that smashes the rock into pieces?" (Jeremiah 23:29) What does a fire do? It destroys everything in its path. Imagine it burning up all disease and each symptom in your body as you speak it over yourself. God's word is smashing the rock of disease in your body into itty bitty pieces! Yahoo! One thing you must get settled is the integrity of God's word and for that I am going to refer you to this teaching[5] or you can search YouTube for

---

[5] "The integrity of God's word" by Kenneth Copeland Ministries: https://www.youtube.com/watch?v=nCDTb7TAQ2c

"The integrity of God's word" by Kenneth Copeland Ministries.

Imagination

"... Nothing will be impossible for them that they have imagined to do." (Genesis 11:6) Get ready for some fun! Visualization puts your subconscious to work to achieve everything you're imagining. Dr. Denis Waitley of the movie 'The Secret,' connected Olympic athletes to biofeedback equipment and had them do their sport only in their mind. This visual motor rehearsal showed that the same muscles fired with the visualization as with when they actually did the sport. The mind didn't know the difference between visualizing and doing. Where the mind goes, the body will follow. Imagine yourself doing the things you cannot physically do currently. When I first tried this, it freaked me out. I was visualizing flexing each foot and bringing my toes toward the ceiling. I have some movement in my feet, but I am not currently able to lift toes or flex my feet upward. As I did this, I could feel the nerves firing! If my eyes were not closed I would have expected to see my feet lifting. The important part of using your imagination to visualize is to engage your emotions to expedite the healing process. Act as if you already have the things that you want. "Therefore, whatever you ask for in prayer, believe you receive it and it will be yours." (Mark 11:24) How would you feel if you were totally healed? Personally, I drop to my knees with my hands up praising God and then I would run across this beautiful country laying hands on the sick on my 'Healing Awareness' tour! Unfortunately, I learned all of this a decade after disease took hold in my body. The disease may have got a head start, but I am taking ground back every day! Every time I get out of bed, I am taking ground back. Every time I visualize, meditate, thank, speak life, laugh, give, and pray, I am taking ground back.

Prayer and meditation

Prayer is powerful if you do it right. I think that God loves it any time we talk to Him, but if you want power you must pray according to what His word says in the Bible. The Bible is what God has already told us. If we pray ignoring what He told us, He can't do much and your prayers won't work. If you're asking God to heal you if it be His will, it is not going to work. You must know what He's already told us about healing. He said that He has already healed you! "Who himself bore your sins in his own body on a tree, that you might be dead to sin and live unto righteousness, by His stripes you were healed." (1 Peter 2:24) Since He has already healed us, there's no reason to ask Him for healing. You've already got it! This is a spiritual truth and to make it manifest in the natural, He tells us to do a variety of things. When we ask for things God told us we have already, He must think, 'if you'd get off your lazy butt and read my word, you would stop begging and start receiving!' Meditation means to think deeply or focus your mind for a period of time. Meditation is not a new age thing, it's a Bible thing. You can focus your mind on pretty much anything. Take five minutes and look at a tree or one scripture. The physical benefits of meditation are numerous. Close your eyes and go to a place that gives you peace. I like green grass. I imagine feeling it on my bare feet. It's nice and cool and soft. It smells amazing. I'm sitting on the grass with my legs crossed. Rolling hills of green grass are before me. "The book of the law shall not depart from thy mouth, but thou shalt meditate therein day and night, that thou mayest observe to do according to all that is written therein: for then thou shalt make thy way prosperous, and then thou shalt have good success." (Joshua 1:8)

Gratitude

I have had to learn to be grateful and the more I do it, the more I want to do it. As I think about all that I have and all the things that I am able to do, thankfulness pours out of me. I thank God for my caregivers every day. I thank God for my dog and my family. I thank God for my living situation. I thank God for my brain and that I am able to tell others how to take good care of me. When you're thankful for things, you get more of them. Coming close to death every single day for over a year totally changes your perspective on life. After that, everything else is a cakewalk. I was so ill and required so much suctioning that I hid the severity of my illness from new caregivers. If they knew what they were getting themselves into, they would never take the job. They would have been too scared and they should have been too scared! There was no one to call for help. The paramedics would have been clueless and if I made it to the hospital alive, they would have surely killed me. We would suction my trachea for up to eight hours! If my caregiver took a break for even a few minutes, I could die because I was having an attack and my lungs were filling at a pace it was hard to keep up with. I did have one caregiver freeze during an attack and walk out of the room. I turned blue and I felt my spirit leaving my body. You'll have to read my first book for the whole story. It took physical strength and endurance to suction for hours. When I think about all the times I peed the bed because I couldn't breathe and my caregiver took too long getting to me, I thank God for my life. I bet survivors of war feel the same way. Many people don't know what real problems are. If I survived that period in my life, I can survive anything. God is merciful.

Adaptability

If you want to survive, you must adapt. I never considered a feeding tube and was very against the idea. However, after a hospital stay being treated for constipation, I was 67 pounds. I immediately called my doctor and initiated the procedure. I never considered a tracheotomy because I had no reason to. I was breathing just fine on my own until one morning I woke up and turned blue. My caregiver called 911 and I was rushed to the hospital only to find out that my blood gasses were at dangerous levels. I had so much carbon dioxide in my blood I should have been dead. If I wanted to live, I had to have a tracheostomy. After being bedbound for three years, I could no longer stand because my feet had contracted. The only way I could get out of bed is to use a hoyer lift. It was overwhelming and scary. I had a choice to make if I ever wanted to leave the bed again. I prayed my way through the fear and anxiety and chose to get out of bed one year ago. Another example of where I adapted to survive is with my defective computer. It was unreliable from day one and would freeze constantly leaving me without a way to call for help. One day, my caregiver was not doing her job and didn't check on me for over an hour. Here's my Facebook post detailing the incident:

> Nutter Butter and I have been side by side going on nine years. One morning last week, my computer froze at ten o'clock and I had no way to call for help. Within a few minutes, I needed suction. The phlegm hitting the plastic of the trach tube woke my dog up. I knew I had to stay calm and keep my breathing relaxed. I

asked God to send in my caregiver before it was too late. An hour later she had still not come in. My dog was sitting at alert and at this point you could hear every breath rattling. He barked once and waited. He barked a second and third time and waited. She came right in and realized the situation. God is faithful and my dog is a hero!

I decided I had had enough of the stupid computer and attached a battery operated doorbell to a pole. This allowed me to kick and ring the bell to call for help when my computer freezes. I use it every single night while I am sleeping just in case my caregiver is not in the room.

I was riding in my van and the caregiver who was driving came to a yellow light, panicked and slammed on the breaks. The caregiver who was riding in the back with me was tossed forward and crashed into the driver's seat. I flew up in the air and my ventilator ripped off. When I landed, I was hanging out of my wheelchair. To prevent this, I made a seat belt for myself that ties me to my wheelchair out of thick upholstery fabric. I would not be here if I hadn't adapted. I don't believe in accommodating disease, but when your back is against the wall, choose life.

Honor and giving

I am sort of a health nut, but I recognize that diet and nutrition is not everything. There are other things that bring you health. Honoring your parents and people in general every chance you get will give you long life. Respecting others is more important than you think. It's good for your soul. Being a giver makes you feel wonderful. Giving is living and takes you out of self-focus. Giving can be financial, things or your time. Giving can be having a neighbor over for dinner, visiting someone in the hospital, or surprising a friend with fresh flowers.

Joy and peace

What gives you joy and peace? I really didn't know. I have been on a search for the things I really enjoy. We get so caught up with the rat race of life and totally forget about our personal happiness and fulfillment. I thought achievement was everything, but it's not always meaningful. I have discovered some things I truly enjoy.

Fresh flowers from your own yard are the coolest thing. Getting rid of things you no longer use is highly enjoyable because it means you get to go shopping. Planning trips to go places I've never been is a blast. I enjoy watching my caregivers experience new things and places. The list goes on and on. A merry heart doeth good like a medicine, but a broken spirit drieth the bones (Proverbs 17:22). As far as peace goes, let's start with some quiet. We all need to have silence, at least fifteen minutes a day. You can make decisions to create peace in your life. Stop being a people pleaser. Eliminate the access that crazy people have to you. If possible, delegate your busy work to others so that you can do the meaningful stuff you enjoy. Set boundaries and standards that give you peace.

CHAPTER THREE

STAND UP FOR YOURSELF AND FIGHT FOR YOUR RIGHT TO PARTY

If you ain't gonna fight for yourself, ain't nobody else gonna honey! Nobody cares about your situation more than you so you cannot expect other people to fight your battles. It's like when you ask everyone else to pray for you when you're not even praying for yourself. I was not always well enough to take a stand. It takes energy and determination. When I stand up for what is right, I am not just doing it for myself, but for those who cannot stand up for themselves and all of those that follow me. I am not talking about the petty stuff. You have to weigh whether or not it's worth your peace to go to bat. I used to be more reserved about making a stink, but I have spent time with the Lord and that gives you quick discernment and boldness. Once I was fighting something or other and asked my caregiver to mail the letter I had typed. She busted out laughing when she saw my letterhead that read, "From the

Offices of Elizabeth Smith". Laugh all you want Millennial Cupcake, because it's from these offices that I sign your check! It's our duty to speak up for justice. Being silent is criminal, cowardly and destroys your own self esteem. Speak up for yourself and others. Don't be such a weenie!

It seems that I have had to fight for pretty much everything. I have fought for many things including: getting on Medicaid, getting my wheelchair repaired, getting a new computer to replace my defective one, getting prescriptions covered by insurance, getting hospital and ambulance bills covered by insurance, ensuring that I am cared for properly every day, keeping a full staff, finding doctors and a hospital that don't violate my right to be heard, finding medical supply companies that will provide good service and fighting pressure sores and respiratory infections every week. I even fight heat rashes on my vagina because my Chihuahua believes he has to be touching it at all times! This list is not conclusive and there are many, many other things! I would like to share a few of my victories with you because they were well earned.

HOA Victory

My Home Owners Association sent the owner of the house I live in letter after letter saying that I was not allowed to park my van in the driveway because it was being stored not driven. I requested a form from the HOA that had my doctor state that it was a medical necessity to park the van in the driveway. It could not be parked in the garage because if for any reason it didn't start, I would be unable to get out of the house because my lift would be blocked. After two years, the HOA gave me approval to park in my driveway!

Pulmonary Victory

I thought I liked my pulmonary doctor, until I had a problem and he wouldn't listen. I had a CAT scan done because I chipped a tooth and thought it was lodged in my throat. The results didn't show a tooth, but it did show that my esophagus was severely deviated because the trach cuff was over inflated. I already had an appointment scheduled with him for my quarterly trach change[6] and was looking forward to discussing the CAT scan results with him. For a video of one of my trach

---

[6] For a video of a trach change when I did them at home, watch this! https://www.youtube.com/watch?v=vjwLqURXLIs

changes when I did them at home, check out the footnote at the end of the chapter!

When we gave him the radiology report, his solution was merely to put less air in the cuff. Sounds good and all, but when your trachea has been stretched for years, that is not practical. He did the trach change and put less air in the cuff. I was farting out of my neck there was so much air escaping around the trach hole! You could hear my voice making sounds! I was not getting full breaths. We told him this was not okay and he said do not add any more air. I told my caregiver to add air so I can breathe and he watched her do it, got mad and left. I cannot believe he was going to leave me gasping for air. When we left the room, we were surrounded by the nurses and someone from administration that looked like they were about 12 years old. They told us that my staff was not allowed to touch me in the procedure room. I have been through this many times and told them that this was a battle they were not going to win. I began looking for a new doctor the next day. Not only did I find a new doctor who listened, he was more than happy to let my staff take care of me. He came up with a real solution to my problem. He suggested getting a longer trach tube so that the cuff would hit the trachea at a different place and allow the stretched area to heal. How smart! Here is the letter I received from the original hospital:

August 20th, 2018

Dear Ms. Smith,

I am writing you as follow up to concerns voiced during your visit on July 12th, 2018, regarding the expectations of care at our hospital. There was question as to what would and would not be permissible during future visits and I would like to offer some clarification and hopefully, some reassurance.

We support the philosophy of Patient and Family-Centered Care. The individual, spiritual, and cultural needs of the patient are supported by welcoming the presence of visitors to the patient. Our visitation policy provides a general framework for creating an environment to welcome patients' family members, significant others, caretakers and guests while ensuring the appropriate medical care, privacy, and safety for patients. The first priority is the care, safety, and privacy of patients, and so visitation must be managed in a manner that promotes physical healing and decreased psychological stress, while also maintaining strict safety standards.

This philosophy also pertains to the care provided to our patients during needed medical procedures, such as the tracheostomy tube change you underwent in July. Although we recognize the personalized expertise of your caregivers, we do maintain that only formally trained and licensed personnel within our facility provide medical assistance for you while in our care; this includes tasks such as suctioning, as well as manipulation of the tracheostomy cuff. The physicians, nurses and technicians are held to strict standards in terms of practice, hygiene and medical equipment use; and the expertise of our staff is confirmed by years of education, competency training and an abundance of experience with patients of all backgrounds and medical histories. Our goal in limiting the provision of medical care to directly employed medical professionals is not to be punitive; it is simply to ensure that you are safe, as well as ensure that the caretakers are safe in the case of an adverse event. Please know that going forward, medical care provided during your procedures will only be provided by our employed medical personnel.

But our priority is also to promote healing and decrease stress. For this reason, we want to reiterate that we will welcome your team of caregivers into the procedural area, when appropriate. Again, with safety being the utmost priority, we will enforce restrictions of one or two caregivers in the procedural area at one time; this is also at the discretion of the medical team conducting the procedure. Our hope is that by inviting your caregivers into the room with you, you will find a sense of comfort. We also recognize that therapeutic communication is extremely important during these stressful times and we are thankful for any assistance they may be willing to provide in this regard. Should you have any questions or concerns prior to your next appointment, please don't hesitate to reach out.

Sincerely, Risk Management

My reply:

Thank you for your emails. I have found a doctor and a facility that are happy to accommodate me and my staff. I will not be returning to your hospital or to your doctor. I have been through this many times before and I am not willing to risk my safety letting people who don't know my communication or how I need to be cared for touch me. I have been hurt several times by hospital staff because they do not know my care. One thing you need to realize is that I have equipment that your staff is not trained on or authorized to use. The Trilogy ventilator and the Respironics cough assist are equipment that your hospital doesn't even own. You are fortunate that my caregivers were there or you would be liable. Elizabeth Smith

(I should have told them I found a doctor that accommodated my dog too! He sat right in my lap during the procedure!)

Technology Victory

I received my second computer that has eye gaze capabilities two and a half years ago. From day one, it would freeze and had many problems. I called technical support almost every day for a while and was told I was doing something wrong. Little did I know that this particular model had problems with software compatibility with its operating system, something I found out 18 months after receiving it. They were paid by Medicare and it was approximately 13k. The company would not take responsibility. My friend Gayle called management at every level and nobody would do anything. I came close to death one morning because the computer froze and I needed suction. I wrote a letter to the tech support manager and told him that I would involve whoever was needed to resolve the situation. I guess he didn't believe me. I filed a report with the attorney general and they did nothing. Gayle called Medicare and they did nothing. We double-teamed them! While she was relentlessly calling VP's at the company, I just happened to watch the documentary 'Gleason.' In the movie they said that they were spending 400k a month to this company to buy devices for people with ALS. I emailed Team Gleason and within one day I received an email from the same manager to whom I sent the letter, saying he was shipping me a brand new computer that day. Bet you'll never forget about me, mister! I'll visit you in your dreams! The victory is so sweet. The following week the president of the company called me from Sweden while on a trip! "Do not avenge yourselves beloved, but leave room for God's wrath. For it is written, vengeance is mine saith the Lord, I will repay." (Romans 12:19) I don't know anything about football and I don't know Steve Gleason, but what his team was willing to do for me was awesome! I don't know his wife either, but from the movie, I love her! I really wish that my husband would have had half the balls to stick it out like she did (proverbial balls, of course).

Wheelchair Repair Victory

I am still in a wheelchair that does not fit me and is extremely uncomfortable. I have owned the wheelchair almost four years, but because I was bedbound for three, it was never worked on. I just fired my wheelchair guy because he had two years and didn't get much done. I would tell him about issues and nothing would happen. In May of this year, I asked him to order an electric hoyer and a shower chair and I found out in September that he had not even submitted the paperwork for approval from Medicaid. You really must stay on these people or you will fall through the cracks! I told him that he was a nice guy, but I was taking my business elsewhere because I need someone who can get things done. He tried to blame it on me somehow (don't they always do that?). That's about 10k he missed out on because he couldn't file paperwork! My new guy is probably tired of me bugging him already. At least he knows that I will not be ignored. He is cute, so I kind of like bugging him!

Soon-to-be Contractor Victory

I hired a contractor to remodel my bathroom in order to make the shower wheelchair accessible. My last shower was over four years ago and I reek, I tell ya! He did my guest bathroom the previous year and did a great job. When he came to do my bathroom, he was a different person. He was very angry every day and acted like it was an inconvenience for him to do the job. Never mind the fact that he was being paid handsomely. I relocated from my room into the office, which was not comfortable for several reasons. He said he would need ten days straight, but he was trying to finish the job for a month and never did. Most days he was gone by one o'clock and took off most weekends. He was rude and yelled at me. My caregivers wanted to wring his neck. He accused me of changing the project and told me to prove that I didn't. I sent him three emails regarding three different things he accused me of changing that proved I had requested it months before. He became furious, turned beat red and walked off the job within two days after receiving my emails. What he left me with is a giant mess. Exposed wiring, cracked and scratched tile, grout covering tile, uneven surfaces, grout missing, crooked tile and a bad paint job are just some of the problems he left, in addition to leaving many things that were originally included in his bid undone. I don't think he knows who he is dealing with! I consider it sport to document my case and recoup my deposit and every penny of the cost of materials – even if I have to represent myself! I am currently filling out the paperwork to go to small claims court and for him to be served. Wish I could be there to see the shock on his face!

Decide beforehand to be the squeaky wheel because if you do, you will get the grease. Who cares if people don't like it, they are not the ones who are in your situation. It is a good thing to have a reputation as someone who has a low bullshit tolerance.

What I mean by 'you have to fight for your right to party' is that some people will always try to push you down because they don't like themselves. They are miserable and want you to be also. You have to get them out of your life. If you're not going to bring something good to the table, you gotta go! Don't be afraid to kick people out of your room, your house and your life. The price is too high to keep dream crushers in your life. The list of people I have kicked out of my house is long. I kicked a home health nurse out because she was pushy and literally told her to get out several times until she left. I have kicked several caregivers out for a multitude of reasons. I kicked an interviewee out because she refused to speak to me directly. I have kicked my own mother out on numerous occasions for crossing the boundaries and bought her a plane ticket home! I can no longer spend time with people who don't respect my wishes. "Better a small meal of vegetables with love than a fattened calf with hatred". (Proverbs 15:17) If someone asks you something that is none of their business, just tell them you're out of the office and will let them know when you return.

CHAPTER FOUR

SELF-EXPRESSION WITH OR WITHOUT A SPEECH GENERATION DEVICE

Part I: Self-Expression With a Speech Generation Device

If someone does not feel heard, it is easy for them to turn inward, withdraw, and shut down. Making your needs known, self-expression and socializing are part of staying healthy. I would be an absolute mess if I didn't have my computer. I am still a mess with it! I am not the kind of person who can just go with the flow. I have 'things to do, people to see and places to go' as my dad would say. I have always envied those people who are just fine with whatever. My caregivers always say that I am always ten steps ahead of them. I am a lot of work, but I am worth it. Talking to someone using a device to speak can be confusing and unfortunately niceties or manners can disappear. Because of the work involved with typing with your eyes, you tend to get to the point quickly. "Would you change the channel dear?" turns into "change channel." I feel there is a need for a guide of some sort to help caregivers, family and friends communicate with someone using a speech generation device. So, here it is!

1. *Have a seat!*

The first thing I would like to say is that you have to dial it down. What I mean by that is if you are talking to someone using a computer to speak, you might as well have a seat and get comfortable because this is going to take a while. When someone is in a hurry and has their pants on fire for an answer and watches every letter I type like they are going to explode if it takes one second longer, I make lots of mistakes because I am trying to hurry and it takes much longer for me to respond than if they just chilled out. Look, I am one of those people who likes to do things as fast as possible and I understand it is partial torture to wait for each letter to be typed out. I am right there with you. Let's not lose perspective though, what a wonderful tool the computer is and just imagine if you did not have it. So, act like the world is not going to end today and chill! Personally, I don't like it when people watch every letter I type and get up in my face. Remember, the computer will speak when I am done typing the sentence. You don't need to be up in my grill yo.

2. *Technology is imperfect*

Keep in mind that technology is not perfect and it has glitches that can make conversation a challenge. There are times when I am not even looking at the computer, but it will catch my eye and start typing and saying things. Sometimes, people will look at me like I'm crazy or like what? You are not making any sense. Okay fine, let's switch places and see how many mistakes YOU make typing with your eyes! It's easy to forget what an effort it is to type with your eyes when someone becomes proficient and you're around them on a daily basis. I have some preprogrammed buttons on my speech screen. The okay button is right next to the clear button so I am always hitting it by accident. If someone is talking, it sounds like I am cutting them off. The tone of the computer is pretty rude and it offends people. It is terrible! If you don't understand that it was a mistake, you just think I am rude. The computer does not always pronounce words correctly so if something sounds weird, please look at the screen. I have a button that says 'stretch feet,' but it sounds like 'scratch feet.'

3. *Chat no more*

Medicare replaces the computer every six years. My first computer was named Lola (by the legendary magical caregiver, Priscilla Martinez) and my current computer I named Laverne. I was very excited to get Miss Laverne over two years ago. Unfortunately, when I received it, it was much more difficult to talk with people. The speed of the typing varies and sometimes it can take up to ten seconds to type one letter. It was extremely disappointing. The company who makes the computer, decided to remove an important feature for conversing. This feature is called the *chat* button. This button allowed you to have two conversations at once without losing anything you had already typed. For example, let's say you were typing a list of things that needed to be done and someone asks you a question. You could hit the chat button and it would clear the screen so you could answer and then go back to your list. Please put it back company! I know you're going to read this and you know who you are. Don't make me come on you like a spider monkey! Now if you have already typed something and someone asks you a question, you pretty much have to lose everything you typed to answer the question unless you speak your list and sound insane. Only if you speak, will you be able to go back and retrieve it. I just found out from my wonderful rep that the chat feature was not removed. I just talked to a tech support guy who was apparently hit upside the head with a dumb stick! Just goes to show you that you have to ask the right person.

4. Save your eyes

Eyes can get worn out quickly if the screen brightness is too high. I set mine to zero because anything more than that burns my eyes and fast. The people at the company who determined the screen brightness obviously weren't the ones using it. At 100% brightness, you cannot even use it as it will burn your eyes to a crisp in less than 5 minutes. Please understand that it is a great effort to type with your eyes. Using abbreviations for things that you need often helps a lot. Here are some abbreviations that I use: S = sheet, H = hands, F = feet and V = vent. I use abbreviations for everything and it saves my eyes. Think about if you had to type out everything you needed in a day and couldn't do anything for yourself. That's many needs and doesn't include conversation. I sometimes will have four interviews in a row. I have most of the buttons preprogrammed, but each person is different and the questions don't all apply. After four interviews, my eyes are toast. If you are a caregiver, please learn abbreviations. It will save you time and their eyes.

5. *Blink or dwell*

Let's talk about the setting on the computer that allows you to select each letter. You can choose from blink or dwell. I'm a blink girl at heart because it tightens your facial muscles and makes you look younger, however when I received Laverne, the blink feature was so difficult to use that I converted to a dwell girl. As a champion blinker, I think that dwell is kind of lame because you stare at the letter until it selects which takes longer, wears your eyes out and has no beauty benefits. Lola had a great blink feature allowing you to blink and move on. The new system doesn't seem to register your blink very well. Are you listening company? Blinking may sound like more work, but I think it's more work to stare and wait.

6. *Misinterpretation*

For me, everything is about doing things with the least amount of eye power. We only have so much energy in a day and I like to conserve it for the fun stuff! If I speak what I have typed, the computer remembers it, but if I don't it does not. This can confuse people for two reasons. Either my caregiver watched me type it and already knows what I'm saying so when I hit the speak button, they may think I am repeating myself when I just want the computer to remember it. This can easily be interpreted as demanding. Or I just typed something completely unrelated to the topic at hand and I speak it so I don't lose it so that I can answer a question and then go back to retrieve what I said later. This can easily be interpreted as bonkers. If you hear something that doesn't make sense, just ask, did you mean to say that or was that a mistake? I will often speak something and keep repeating it on accident because my eyes are catching the eye sensors. If you don't understand how things work, you will be so confused. I am misunderstood often!

7. *Alignment*

The eye gaze alignment has to be just right or nothing works right. While I am sleeping, I shift and wake up to find my calibration is no longer working right and the letters the computer is selecting are not the ones I want to select! This can turn me into a three year old pretty quickly! When I am on the bedpan (which I am entirely too sexy for) it pushes my body up so that my eyes no longer reach my computer and I have to use other forms of communication. Aligning the eye gaze sensors up perfectly and calibrating them takes time and bites the bullet. It can be frustrating when you have something urgent to say. I will cry and cry if it's in the middle of the night because I just want to go back to sleep. Let's be real, it's total bondage to be chained to a machine! And yes, I do sleep with it right in front of my face every night and it is a challenge to adjust my eyes to the bright light if I need help.

8. *It operates with my eyes, not smoke signals from my rear!*

It seems like no matter how many times we tell new caregivers not to block the eye gaze sensors, they still do it. They will ask me a question and then hold their hand or arm in front of the sensor. When they do this, I just stare at them wondering how long it will take them to realize that I cannot answer until they move. Many never realize it and just think I'm weird for staring at them. If you're doing something that requires you to block the computer, please watch the person's face. If they look like they are in distress or like they are trying to tell you something, MOVE! This also applies to when people are showing me things. If they hold it right in front of the computer, it will catch my eyes and start typing things and saying things. When you show something you will want to hold it above or to the side of the computer. When we suction, the sensors catch my eyes and wreak all sorts of havoc on the internet that I have to go back and fix later. When I am typing furiously trying to say something urgent and someone reaches across my computer screen to pick up a piece of lint or hair, I want to scream! That is the same thing as if you were talking and I interrupted you to pick a piece of lint off your shirt. Is the lint really more important than letting me finish?

9. *Hold your horses!*

If you want to help someone, you have to know what they need first. While I appreciate a person who is eager to help, you have to wait until I finish typing! It very easy to assume you know what I am going to say and then start doing it and you're wrong! Just chill. For example, if I type 'h' but I am not done yet and my caregiver starts adjusting my hands, then I type a 'p' after the 'h,' 'hp' is short for heating pad. You're doing something that I didn't even want. If you would have just waited one more second, you would have known exactly what I wanted. Basically in your effort to help, you're not really helping at all. Patience is a virtue. Letting people finish what they are going to say is important. When you're using a device to speak, it's rare that people let you finish your sentence. Sometimes it's not a big deal, but other times it is very frustrating. When I am dealing with an eager beaver, I will describe where I want something done before I tell them what they are doing so they have to let me finish. For example, if I say that I have a hair on my face, I don't want someone to just start randomly touching my face all over. Instead, I will type the location first. Right lower forehead I have a hair. If you're overly eager you can cause extra work for both of us!

10. *Tone of voice*

Remember that you are talking to a computer voice, not your person's voice! Even if the person is using their own voice through a voice bank on the device, the tone is not under their control! The tone of the voice is often offensive. The voice I use can sound really mean. I used to use a child's voice but Alexa, my Amazon Echo, would not respond to it so I switched. If I type the word 'what' without a question mark, get ready for the rudest 'what' on the planet. People get so mad as if I am the one being rude! I recommend naming the device just so you can tell it to shut up! My caregivers are always telling Laverne to zip it. If you're sentimental and miss your person's voice, I understand. It is rough. Just never forget that the tone of voice may or not reflect the feelings behind the words.

11. *Safety*

As we know, technology doesn't work 100% of the time. Caregivers, please continue to check on your people often. There are days when my computer freezes up to twenty times a day and I am unable to call for help. There are many other things that would cause someone to not be able to call for help, such as: sunlight beaming, reflection blocking the eye gaze sensors, the computer stand getting kicked and moving the computer away from eye reach, if a chubby Chihuahua sits on your chest, and if someone is coughing (tough to cough with your eyes open). If possible, have a backup system to call for help. Battery operated doorbells are a great solution.

Sunlight is a big problem for being able to use the eye gaze. If the sun shifts, it creates a huge glare and you can't see what you're typing. Once again, this was not a problem with Lola. The company has changed the screen to a very glossy one. The older screen was dull and wasn't affected by light half as much. There are times I literally have to sit in the dark to be able to communicate!

12. *Custom pages*

Custom pages are a wonderful way to save eye power for things you will be saying every day. Here's a list of some of my custom pages just to give you ideas: Alexa, comfort, exercise, interviews, funny sayings, speak to the mountain, praise, prophecy and scripture. With the Alexa page I can turn lights on and off, find out the outdoor temperature, hear a news report and play my favorite artists like Dolly Parton. The interview page makes the process efficient. I am able to conduct a full interview in less than 45 minutes! I have fun with the funny sayings page, especially in public. I like to go to a store and say things like, 'clean up on aisle four' and 'ba dunk dunky dunk' in my trunk'. I love to speak powerful scriptures over myself and tell symptoms to hit the road in Jesus name!

12. *The uhhh button*

When I want someone to stop what they are doing and don't have the time to type it out, I hit the 'uhhh' button. Everyone stops in their tracks. This is a great tool that works well and I suggest adding it to your custom buttons on your speak page. My custom buttons are: Yes, uhhh, sukilicious, suction, thanks girl, no, please, not sure, okay and Alexa play.

13. *Relationships*

My husband used to have a love hate relationship with Lola. He wanted me to use it when he couldn't understand me, but he always thought I was ignoring him when I was typing. You cannot keep firing off questions if you ever want an answer! I would be typing to answer his first question and he would ask four more! Then he would say that I was ignoring him as I was busy typing. You have to learn patience just as the person using the device had to if you want to maintain your relationship. It is weird and slow to speak to someone using a device, but if you allow that get in the way of your relationships you are just letting the disease win. I think it is more difficult for older generations to understand how it all works. My parents will say something to me and will both be halfway down the hallway by the time I am able to comment. When you are speaking to someone, you may want to glance at the screen to see if they are on the speak page. I will be on my email typing away and someone will try to have a conversation with me, but I don't hear much of it and I cannot reply because I am not on the speak page. It's a good idea to ask them to let you know when it is a good time to talk if you want to be heard.

It is my understanding that the original company who made Lola merged with another company and the conglomerate is manufacturing the current devices. My life would be hell without a way to express myself and I am extremely grateful for my computer as I am in my ninth year of using one. I don't know how many employees of the original company are still around, but they need to work on the current devices! The older versions were far superior. When it comes to web navigation, it was much easier. There was no gaze selection and it was wonderful because your eyes controlled the curser. I wrote my first book with Lola and had to stop using her because you could barely see what you were selecting anymore the selector was so dim. The company doesn't repair devices that old or I would still be using her. She never froze and was very reliable. My opinion is that the new devices come with way too much software on them and it bogs down the whole system. There's software on mine that I will never use. Xbox? Cortana? Skype? Facebook? Cortana is a pain and can't be uninstalled. It is always popping up when I don't want it to. I thank the company for making these devices and I highly recommend that you let the employees of the original company take over the programming and let people download their own software if they want it instead of putting it on the devices automatically.

Part II: Self-Expression Without a Speech Generation Device

You will not always have your device with you so you need a backup form of communication. If you don't have a speech generation device, don't worry! You will be just fine. With facial cues and the ABC's you can do anything if you don't give up.

The first thing you want to determine is your signal for "yes" and "no." I blink for "yes" and just stare for "no." Once you figure out your signs for "yes" and "no," you're well on your way to talking up a storm!

Using yes or no questions sounds easy, but you really have to think sometimes. A yes or no question cannot have the word OR in it. If there is more than one option, you need to ask each one separately and then wait for each answer. A yes or no question cannot have a double negative in it. For example, did you NOT want that? If they answer yes or no, you still don't know the answer.

If the person needs to tell you something that cannot be done with yes or no questions, you can use the ABC's. I mouth the letters 'ABC' to let my caregivers know I need to spell something out using the ABC's, but you can use any cue you want. There is also a letter board that you can make and point to the letters, but who wants to have to find the board every time you have something to say? The caregiver will say the alphabet, separating each letter and the person will blink on the letter. This doesn't have to be slow. In fact, you can get really fast after a while. Use your abbreviations! After each letter, the caregiver needs to repeat it to confirm that it is the correct letter. Let's say the word you are spelling is 'dog'. You will need to say, "d? d-o? d-o-g?" Always repeat the letters you have so far because one wrong letter and you have to start over. If the letter is after the letter m, I will close my eyes letting my caregiver know that they can start at the letter m instead of starting at the beginning of the alphabet. If I am able to mouth any letters, I will do that and it speeds up the process. I can mouth the letters f, o, m, and s pretty well. You can also use a letter and eye movement combination. If I mouth the letter s and look to the left or right, it means 'move my shoulders.' If I mouth the letter s and look at your shirt, it means 'fix my shirt.' If I mouth the letter s and look up, it means 'sheet up.' If I mouth the letter s and look at my computer, it means 'go to settings.'

One thing I need to mention is that it's difficult to hold your eyes open without blinking the whole alphabet, so I will blink several times when it is the right letter. This distinguishes a natural blink from the signal blink. When you get really good, you two don't even need to talk. It is like a well-choreographed ballet. The caregiver can also use signals too and it's kind of neat when they do because we are speaking the same language! One of my caregivers uses signals to fix my shirt. She uses a different hand motion for each part of the shirt and I blink yes or no. It has taken something that I used to dread and made it fun! One useful thing to use if someone is coughing or you have no idea what they need is to say, "look at me if you need xyz". This is a clear way to find out.

When I mouth letters, it looks like I am angry. I know this because of people's reaction. It is an extreme effort to mouth letters! Sometimes I am sweating bullets as I often have to repeat what I am saying several times. Sometimes I bite my lips and tongue and bleed. Sometimes I hit my teeth together and it makes a terrible grinding sound that makes my caregivers cringe. Communicating without speaking is not easy and takes much patience, but you do what you need to do!

CHAPTER FIVE

IF YOU WANNA LIVE, YOU GOTTA POOP!

Pooping is like a box of chocolates, you never know what you're going to get. I suffered for years in this area and I really hope you can learn from my mistakes. I am happy to say that after years of being constipated, I now have a BM just about every day and thank God for each precious turd!

Today, I take a half a cap of Miralax daily and I use a butt douche. If I drink enough water, I don't even need the Miralax! What is a butt douche? Great question! It is a sex toy I discovered while shopping online for something safer and less invasive than the standard bucket and PVC tubing used for enemas. I absolutely have zero curiosity about what people do with it and why it is considered a sex toy. I had been using the standard enema for years with soap suds until a caregiver was a bit too rough inserting the tube and severed a blood vessel, causing me to lose so much blood I needed a transfusion and staples. That was a party, let me tell ya!

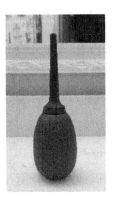

I had tried Miralax before, but it was too large of a dose and caused a constant flow that was unmanageable. I am so glad I was willing to try it again, because I can be stubborn. A half a cap of Miralax is the right amount for my body, but you will have to play around to find what works for you. For the butt douche, I put eight ounces of hot tap water into a container, spray a tiny bit of peppermint Castile liquid soap until I see bubbles, and then pour it into the douche bulb. I use coconut oil to lubricate the tip, insert one or two inches and squeeze! One or two douches usually does the trick. If the bedpan gets too full of liquid to remove it safely, we use a 60 ml syringe supplied by the feeding tube company to suck up the excess fluid and put it in a container to flush in the toilet. If you don't have a syringe, I guess you could use a turkey baster or something. This whole process could easily be done over a toilet if you have long enough arms. This method is very safe, easy, natural and painless! I love it! I recommend this method for anyone who struggles with constipation. I am pretty sure the hospital doesn't use a sex toy for anything, but they should!

I originally learned about the soap suds enema when I was in the hospital preparing for a colonoscopy. I tried my best to drink all of their stupid Go Lytley (should be called Barf Lytley) and failed, so they did a soap suds enema. They also used castile soap that is all natural and can be found at Walmart. I had never heard of this before and loved the idea because I didn't have to take pills, suppositories or drink anymore crap!

The old hanging bucket method with the PVC tubing works. However, unless you have a soft tip for the end of the tubing and are very careful about measuring how far it is inserted, I would not take the chance. At one point we were inserting eight or more inches! This is not safe even though every nurse said it was. I get the same results with the butt douche inserted one or two inches! Listen, when I had that torn blood vessel, it was a three day hospital stay. Please learn from my mistake!

Before I learned about the soap suds enema, I was in poop hell. I was so constipated and impacted that my ureters were squished and I wasn't able to urinate. In order to urinate, my caregiver had to reach into my rectum with a finger and remove the poop. I am not talking about digital stimulation here. I had to call a nurse several times to come to the house and use a catheter for relief. When I was hospitalized for constipation, they put me under anesthesia while a nurse removed the poop manually and inserted a catheter. To their shock and amazement, I completely filled the two-liter urine bag! When I woke, they showed me the bag and I said, "I told you I had to pee!"

During this difficult time of my life, I tried many things to relieve my issues. I tried magnesium citrate (two bottles of the clear liquid in a row), which should have blown my back door clear off, but did nothing. I tried Lactulose but it made me extremely nauseous to the point I stopped eating. Senna pills had the same effect. Suppositories had no effect, not even the Magic Bullet I ordered online. I tried teas like Smooth Move and Get

Regular and they didn't work. Fiber powders are not a good idea when you are not moving your body and only made things worse. I drank Epsom salt mixed with water, and gagged and heaved. The only thing that had any effect was eating a dozen kiwis, but to rid myself of the impaction I would have had to eat hundreds! I was so impacted that I was beyond the help of most remedies. In fact, the feces were so hard that it tore my rectum and I started hemorrhaging. You do not want to know the pain of tearing your pooper shooter! I am thankful for the hemorrhage because otherwise, I would not have gone to the hospital and would not have learned about the soap suds enema. I had lost a significant amount of weight and felt like I was trying everything. Thank God for the soap suds enema!

CHAPTER SIX

HOW TO USE MEDICAL EQUIPMENT FOR SURVIVAL

Feeding Tube

The first medical device I got was my feeding tube in 2012. I was very against it until I got down to 67 pounds and knew how dangerous that was. How did I lose so much weight? Let's just say that I had lots of help. One night I was sitting on the toilet for hours and this particular turd, whom I will call fat Albert, was really putting up a fight. I finally told my husband that I needed some help. We called the ambulance because fat Albert was halfway in and halfway out and we were not sure how to get me in the car. He was in the car business so we always had fancy cars and weren't about to let fat Albert take a cruise! This was my first hospital experience and if I knew what was going to happen, I would have never gone. They gave me a chemical enema, the kind that they mix and put in a container that is connected to your butt with a hose. Two medical assistants administered it. One was in training and the other seemed very unsure of herself. They gave me enough laxative to kill a cow. They put a diaper on me even though I am not incontinent. What happened for the next few hours was like something out of the movie 'The Exorcist.' Most unfortunately, my husband was with me and witnessed the fecal demons aborting my body. My whole body was contorting. I was vomiting. I believe this scared the ever living shit out of him too. It would not surprise me one bit if this is the night he made the decision to emotionally depart our marriage. In sickness and health, unless the fecal demons start flying! What a nightmare. Because they left me in the diaper, I developed a severe kidney infection. I don't know what they gave me, but it had to have been an overdose. The monkeys pulled me to my feet thinking that I could walk to my wheelchair five feet away and you will have to read the whole story in the chapter 'Beware of Hospitals and Facilities.' At this point and time it took me about two hours to eat one meal because I had to be careful not to choke. I was dehydrated and it took me all day to drink 16 ounces of tea. I designed a bib (that I sold in my business) to hold the cup and allow me to drop my head and sip from a straw. I wore it all day long, every day. Of course they were cute, so that helped the situation tremendously! All of this happened over one lousy turd! If you're constipated, for God's sake, please exhaust every effort to get the poop out at home (see the previous chapter if you haven't already for ideas)!

After the procedure, I had a wonderful nurse who told me that I could blend just about anything and put it in the tube. I'm grateful for that nurse because I have heard that some people are told that they cannot eat real food and have to settle for the formula. I tried the formula for a while, but I couldn't tolerate the smell. Formula is very convenient, but if you look at the label it's full of preservatives, artificial ingredients and sugar. I still ate by mouth, but when I got tired I finished my meal through the tube. Refried beans, stuffed shells, fish and chips, PF Chang's and anything I wanted, all went through the tube. It wasn't until years later that I got serious about nutrition.

If you have a feeding tube, it's time to take full advantage of not having to taste healthy things that are disgusting. First things first, get hydrated. It took forever for me to drink by mouth and drinking was speedy by tube! That was a big advantage for me. I am going to give you some tips on putting real food through a feeding tube because sometimes it's not easy. You will need a good blender and food processor, a coffee grinder, a mortar and pestle and some big muscles. The nurse suggested a Vitamix, but that is expensive so I am looking for a pre-owned one. I use a Cuisinart and a blender that has to be replaced periodically. People always ask if I am able to taste food as it is going into my stomach and oddly enough, I can taste peanut butter, green apples, and garlic.

Before I went vegetarian I would cook large quantities of food and freeze it. I roasted two whole chickens which only blended down to twelve cups and added raw frozen spinach. I baked twenty sweet potatoes at a time, blended and then froze them. It was a lot of work for my caregivers and was very time consuming. This is why I came up with Café G: the first feeding tube-friendly take out franchise. Unfortunately, the state of Colorado doesn't allow you to prepare food in your home to sell and getting a commercial kitchen is a cost that I am not able to manage at this point. I did have one customer whom I gave free food to as I was developing the idea. She died. Not because she ate my food (I see you smiling!). This made me wonder about the viability of this business, however, according to the people at Feeding Tube Awareness, almost 200,000 procedures are performed each year. With millions of people having feeding tubes, I believe this business could really work. It can be extremely difficult to get the food ground down fine enough to go through the tiny hole at the end of the feeding extension tube. I have had many machines start smoking. I am going to share with you my first menu to give you an idea of what you can do.

Welcome to Café G!
Why give up good food just because you have a G tube? Why eat the formula made by big corporations that are full of preservatives and chemicals? You deserve better! Our meals are delivered frozen to your door and designed to be given through bolus feeds using a 60 ml syringe. Treat your tummy right!

Many disorders are hyper-metabolic making it difficult to even maintain weight let alone gain it. I'm 5 ft 5" tall and have always been thin (105 lbs), however, when I got my G-tube I weighed 67 pounds! I tried the formula but it made me nauseous. Since I have been eating real food I have become... well, let's just say that none of my old clothes fit! Our food is high calorie, high fat (the good fats) and high protein and jam packed with nutrition! Low fat available upon request. Our meals are also available for strictly mouth eaters too, unblended!

MENU

Tuna Nicoise - White albacore tuna (24 oz), white beans, boiled eggs, black olives and extra virgin olive oil
* Gluten Free and Dairy Free
6 cups $19.99 (approximately 24 syringes)

Chicken a la Kale - Baked chicken, sautéed kale, sweet potatoes and extra virgin olive oil
* Gluten Free and Dairy Free
6 cups of chicken and kale $14.99   6 cups sweet potatoes $14.99   (approximately 48 syringes)

Victoria's Real Secret - All natural peanut butter, non-dairy Kefir (probiotics!) and blueberries
*Gluten Free and Dairy Free
6 cups $14.99 (approximately 24 syringes)

Pork Hawaii Five-0 – Slow-cooked pork roast in crushed pineapple, mashed potatoes (made with 2% milk and real salted butter), baby peas and extra virgin olive oil
6 cups pork roast $24.99   6 cups mashed potatoes and peas mixed $14.99 (approximately 48 syringes)

Vegetarian Lentil Stew - Lentils, carrots, onions, celery, raisins and extra virgin olive oil
* Gluten Free and Dairy Free
6 cups $14.99 (approximately 24 syringes)

BUILD YOUR OWN QUICHE COMING SOON!

Serving Instructions

Supplies needed: 60 ml syringes, 24 inch extension feeding tube, a placemat (or something to protect the surrounding area) and a fabric towel (or ten, if you're a beginner).

Typically, you don't have to clip the extension tube because the food is too thick to run out. Plus, clipping causes kinks in the tube that will become an annoying fly on your overworked, out of time ass.

DO NOT let go of where the syringe connects to the extension tube. Food will shoot halfway to the moon! Until you build some endurance, you may have to use your shoulder or knee to push, but keep it close, it's connected to an organ for heaven's sake! And don't say it's too hard, you can do this. I suppose if you're a real weinershnitzel you can water it down.

Trouble Shooting

No pain, no gain - but well worth it!

If you get a clog and you will, these are some things to do:

- [ ] Is it clipped? Duh.
- [ ] Pull back and then push on the syringe.
- [ ] Look for the block and squeeze the tube with your fingers.
- [ ] Take the tube off and use a toothpick to dislodge.
- [ ] If all else fails get a new extension tube and kick the dog.
- [ ] Never just push as hard as you can because when it finally goes through it hurts! Ask me how I know.
- [ ] Pipe cleaners can also be useful.

How to Eat

People are not gerbils and therefore, we do not 'feed.' We eat.

Push and pause just like you do when you chew your food. Take at least a few minutes to finish one syringe. Five minutes is ideal for one syringe. Stop pushing for any coughing, yawning, sneezing and hiccups. Four syringes equal one cup, but remember this food has been blended so it's much more than that. Body position needs to be in at least a thirty degree incline to avoid reflux. It's helpful to put the syringes of food in a container of hot water, otherwise do not heat. Pulling some water up in empty syringes aids the cleaning process. Lubricating the stoppers of the syringe in olive oil can ease with the pushing, you old goat!

The list of what I eat every day is below. From looking at it, you would think that I should be leaping tall buildings in a single bound. Being vegetarian has its advantages because there is no cooking. I switch back and forth from vegan to vegetarian and sometimes I eat liver too. This diet is pricey. Organic raw cashews and almonds are easily over nine bucks a pound and ten pounds of organic chicken livers is over forty dollars!

2 organic bananas

1 avocado

2 cups of organic kale

1 organic apple

5 stalks of organic cilantro

1/2 cup of organic raw almonds

1/2 cup of organic raw cashews

4 tbsp of coconut milk

3 tbsp of hemp seeds

3 tbsp of chia seeds

2 tbsp of wild caught sockeye salmon

2 garlic cloves

1/2 tsp of acacia powder (prebiotic)

1 serving of organic acai powder

1 serving of organic goji powder

1 tsp of organic turmeric powder

1 crushed iron pill

1 crushed B-12 pill

1 punctured and drained fish oil pill (vitamin d)

1 lion's mane mushroom capsule

In addition to the diet above (which is made into a smoothie every day) I take two Dr. Axe soil-based organism probiotics (yes, I eat dirt!) and a half a cap of Miralax. I take no medication other than two nebulizer treatments twice a day. I also eat eight ounces of fermented sauerkraut or vegetables when we have it made. I'm told it's the best kraut! I believe this is the right diet for me at the moment and I am not against meat. If our country continues to eat meat and dairy products that are full of antibiotics, we will continue to be a sick nation. As Dr. Axe says in the video at the end of this chapter, research shows that pesticides cause brain disfunction. We really don't know all of the things that pesticides cause. Research over decades shows that organic produce has significantly more antioxidants and disease fighting benefits.

Here's a list of produce that does and doesn't need to be organic, according to Dr. Axe:

The dirty dozen (needs to be organic):
apples, celery, peaches, bell peppers, kale, cherries, lettuce, nectarines, grapes, carrots, pears, and strawberries.
The clean fifteen (doesn't need to be organic):
pineapple, mangoes, papaya, watermelon, kiwi, sweet potatoes, tomatoes, broccoli, cabbage, asparagus, avocados, eggplant, onions, sweet peas and sweet corn.

Tracheostomy

The tracheostomy is the second medical device I had installed into my body in 2014 and I was in rehab for 35 days in the high alert area. As I mentioned in chapter two, I never even thought about a tracheostomy, but I woke up and turned blue because my blood gas levels were so bad. When I was being monitored in the hospital before the procedure, a pulmonologist told me she had never seen someone with so many oral secretions. What can I say? I'm juicy! It has become a common occurrence for doctors' jaws to drop over some aspect of my body. If you look at the pictures of me on Facebook, it would be easy to think that I don't fight serious issues on a daily basis. Just because I never talk about them doesn't mean I don't have any. My caregivers help me fight severe symptoms every day. During an outpatient hospital procedure, I contracted pseudomonas, a dangerous bacteria that as far as I know, I still test positive for to this day. This bacteria causes the volume of secretions to be very high. Here is a picture of the machine with my oral secretions from a twenty four hour period. It has a blue iridescent hue to it from the pseudomonas. That is a lot of spit! Most days, my jaw and facial muscles are sore from working it up.

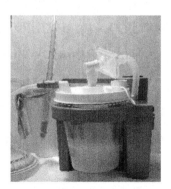

After being on heavy duty antibiotics for over a year including a nebulizer antibiotic that cost over 5k a month (that my poor dad paid for), I found a doctor who told me that the bacteria was colonized and I would have it for life (doubt it buddy!). He took me off the antibiotics and started nebulizer treatments instead that have been very effective.

Before pseudomonas, trach care was simple and consisted of cleaning the dried secretions from around the trach. Now, trach care is the most challenging part of my care. Mucus pours from the trach and a fresh gauze often lasts less than five minutes. Nebulizer treatments two to four times a day has helped to reduce the suctioning from over 100 times a day to less than 30 times a day. When I drink water, it's difficult to manage. If I go out, I make sure to not drink any water beforehand or during. Having a trach is like going from having no allergies to having terrible allergies. I have the feeling that I am going to sneeze all the time. Having a trach also limits your sense of smell and taste because there is no air flow through your nose or mouth. There is a psychological adjustment when you cannot breathe out of your nose or mouth. A sense of deep panic sets in as your brain says there is something very wrong here. This took years to overcome.

If you have a pulmonary condition of any kind, with or without a trach, there is one machine you must have. The Cough Assist made by Respironics saves my life every day and it can be seen in action in the video at the end of the chapter. I received it years before I got the trach and used it with a mask over my mouth. Now, it fits right on my trach. It shoves a huge breath of air into your lungs and then sucks it out along with the junk that is hindering your breathing. While I am drinking water and the cough assist is on, secretions are forced out through my mouth like a waterfall pouring down my face and neck which is a real blast to clean up. (Being my caregiver is not a glamorous job!) The mask takes lots of practice so don't give up. This is a powerful machine! It is not uncommon for it to pull out a ton of mucus that goes all over my bed and my shirt, but better out than in! It is for this reason I am not interested in dating at the moment. Could you imagine? Picture it on Farmers.com: *If you have a thing for mucus, I'm your gal!* That is disgusting!

Another piece of equipment that is nice to have is a SmartVest. It's a vest that shakes your torso violently and keeps mucus from sticking to the lungs.

This is a picture of Lizette. She helps us train new people on how to suction and work with the trach. "Hi, I'm Lizette, got a cigarette?"

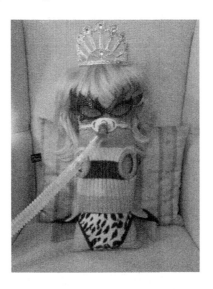

Next is a picture of a trach tube. Not all trach's have a cuff, but mine does. The cuff is the round piece that is inflated along the white tube that goes into my trachea. The cuff keeps the oral secretions from going down into the lungs and keeps it in place. There is a valve that you can attach to the trach that allows you to talk. I tried it in the hospital, but did not tolerate it because the cuff has to be deflated and there were too many secretions. The round inflated piece at the end of the cord stays on the outside, usually in my shirt. This is how it is inflated or deflated using a 10 ml syringe.

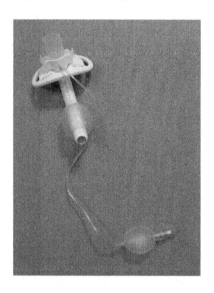

Because I require constant trach care, there are always arms, hands and fingers touching me. There are times when I do not tell anyone that I need a new gauze because I don't want to be touched. This can be claustrophobic. I would rather let mucus run down my chest than to have arms jab my nose, hands bumping into my face and boobs squashing me sometimes. It's one of those things that I cannot think about because I will go insane. There are many things that I cannot allow myself to think about. Another aspect of my care that is constant is the changing of the ventilator pieces that connect it to my trach. Because the air coming through the ventilator is warm, condensation collects inside the plastic cylinders when the room air is cooler than the ventilator air. The condensation will drip into my trachea and cause violent coughing. It's just like when you swallow and water or whatever you're drinking goes down the wrong pipe. This happens 24/7 and requires my caregivers to change the pieces constantly. When the air conditioning is on, the pieces can get wet in less than 5 minutes!

People ask me if suctioning hurts and the answer is no. If it's done properly, there is no pain. If someone goes too deep and hits my carina, THAT hurts. The carina is the cartilage above where the trachea branches off and goes to the right or left bronchi. Suctioning is time consuming and interrupts whatever you are doing. Sometimes I will type an email during suctioning, it's so boring.

I have four suction machines, two for home and two for travel. The ventilator I use is made by Trilogy. I am grateful for the machinery, but I will not need it forever. I am currently working with my doctor checking gas levels to work towards weaning off the vent. It is a big thing to take on, but not for God!

Stretching and exercise

Stretching and exercise is an important part of survival. Because I am not walking, the tendons and ligaments want to shorten. It is crucial to stretch in order to prevent this and other problems. At the end of this chapter I will share a video of my leg stretches[7] and no, I am not a contortionist in the Cirque du Soleil! Stretching is painful and I don't want to do it, but I am committed to my health.

Working out to the best of my ability makes me happy. I do what I can do and don't think about what I can't do. Getting my heart pumping any way I can clears my head and has physical and psychological benefits. I get lazy like anyone else and don't want to work out, but I always feel better when I do. I do butt lifts, knee squeezes, leg lifts, abdominal crunches and holding my legs in the air. A video of my leg lifts is at the end of this chapter. In the video, I do over one hundred lifts but my typical routine is a minimum of 400 leg lifts. That may

---

[7] https://www.youtube.com/watch?v=tmyDVFBmfFQ&t=67s

seem like a lot for someone with my diagnosis, but I have not even scratched the surface of my capability. At 500 leg lifts, I am doing okay - so I know I can do more. A wedge, as shown in the video, is a wonderful tool for exercise or for changing your position in bed.[8]

It's fun to challenge myself just like when I was running. Walking is something I also love and would walk for hours on the beach into the next township or two. One story my mother enjoys telling is when she came to visit me in Florida. I took her for a walk on the beach. I didn't tell her where or how far we were going because I didn't know myself. We walked passed a couple of towns before we turned around. At the turn around point, she asked to take a break. She was not happy. She claimed I drank all her water and I never brought any on these excursions. She didn't wear proper footwear and her foot was bleeding. She spotted an RV with Missouri plates (where we are from) and wanted to ask them to rescue her, but I wouldn't let her because it was too embarrassing. She was very upset with me. On the many miles home I was getting yelled at. When we finally arrived at the condo, her toes looked like raw

---

[8] https://www.youtube.com/watch?v=VpE23kvwGLE

hamburger. She thought it would be a good idea to use the jacuzzi to alleviate all her aching muscles. We went out to the jacuzzi and unfortunately, she was so exhausted that she missed the first step and fell head first into the water! That was definitely not her day. Twenty years later and she still talks about it. In California, I either walked from Santa Monica through Venice to Marina Del Rey for my short walk or through Malibu to Zuma Beach for a long walk. If you know Los Angeles, that is a long way!

Symptoms

I'm going to list some of the symptoms I fight just so you understand that I am actively fighting every day: hyper reflexes, spasticity, foot contractures that cause toe sores, extreme volumes of oral and tracheal secretions, hot skin spots, severe flushing, hives from heat, scalp soreness and heat rash, muscle knots throughout, hyper extension of hip from the bedpan, punctured ear drums and spine pain from protruding vertebrae. That's just off of the top of my head! As I wrote that list, I was thinking that I know it could be so much worse and for that I am grateful.

The first time I experienced the full force of spasticity, I bit my bottom lip so hard and for so long that I drew blood where each tooth had been from canine to canine. One winter I did not use the heater much because I was hot. My caregivers wore their coats, hats, gloves and scarves. I was so hot and miserable that I let the temperature in the house drop below 60 and all of my pet fish died. All visitors know they need to bring warm clothes and layer up or they will freeze. We have washed my hair and seen steam come off my head.

CHAPTER SEVEN

HOW FAMILY, FRIENDS AND CAREGIVERS CAN HELP

The first thing I have to say about family and friends supporting someone with a terminal diagnosis is that you have to control your grief. In the first several years after my diagnosis, people would come to visit me and would grieve right in front of me as if I was already dead. Not only was this confusing, but I had enough to deal with emotionally and to then try to understand their grief was overwhelming. I was still alive! These days, now that I am on a ventilator and use equipment to survive, I can understand that it might be hard to see me, especially if you knew me before the diagnosis. Friends and family, you have to be strong! Have faith! The body is not who we are anyhow. We are spirits that live in a body. Our bodies are merely containers for our spirits. This is not the time to break down and cry, do that in privacy. Things could change in a New York minute and you could die before them! Do your best to treat them normally. There is nothing wrong with saying you are there for them but please don't talk about losing them. Help them fight! Keep it light. Honor them by continuing to visit and by not disappearing like many people do. Not knowing what to say is not a good enough reason to stay away. Suck it up and just say hi. Talk about the future. Make plans for next year.

Faith helps a great deal and I don't mean talking about going to be with the Lord. I once had a visiting nurse who was ridiculous. During his first visit he spoke in a very soft, sad voice and asked me if life was worth living. I looked around wondering who he was talking to! I thought, "maybe not for you bozo, but my life is great!" I hate sympathy! Compassion and sympathy are two different things. It's totally fine to show your love, but the second you start saying things like, "awe, I'm sorry sweetie" and start petting them like a dog, you are not helping! If you want to help say things like, "you got this! You're strong!" and make them laugh! "Oh child, you're going to rock a bald head!" Or whatever! If you are ooey-gooey with the sympathy and tears, they will not look forward to your visits.

Caregivers, the first thing you need to do is learn your job. Learn how the equipment works and how to do everything in the most sanitary ways as possible. I have found that people do not like to wash their hands in general. I won't let my caregivers touch me after they arrive until they wash their hands. I am always asking if they washed their hands. It shocks me when new caregivers are not really paying attention during training. Everything we show them is important and I would not want to be the one responsible if something happened. People are so afraid to hurt me and I used to tell them that they couldn't hurt me unless they didn't respond to my call for suctioning. Well, my entire viewpoint of that has changed thanks to a new caregiver who did some things that I never imagined could happen. She seemed to be catching on during training or I would never have allowed her to be on her own. The first time she helped to put me in the wheelchair, she attached the ventilator without an exhalation valve. I didn't notice that I was only inhaling for a couple minutes. It hit me all of the sudden and I felt like I was going to pass out. My computer was not adjusted correctly and I couldn't tell the caregivers what was happening. By the time they figured it out, I was not okay. The carbon dioxide was building up in my system. It could have been a sad day, but God! One of my daily prayers is for protection from human error. A couple of days later, I was using the cough assist and that same caregiver couldn't take it off! It was attached to my trach and just kept going cycle after cycle. I was giving her the cue to take it off, but she just couldn't get it. The next week was the final straw. She was lowering me into my wheelchair using the hoyer and didn't shut the valve off when I landed so it kept lowering. The steel bars were digging into my skin on my chest and arms. The other caregiver had to drag it off of me and it was still lowering! You must pay attention to what you're doing because there is too much at stake.

The next thing caregivers can do to help is to stop complaining. There have been days when I feel like a shrink. One person comes in talking about every little problem in their life and every little physical ailment they have and then the next person comes in and does the same thing. Sometimes I think they need their own caregiver! I care and want to know if something major is going on, but sometimes it's just too much. It's also kind of insensitive. Complaining to someone who has seen more pain and suffering than they could imagine. I need to know if they are having trouble doing aspects of the job, but I am sorry, I don't want to know every detail of what you just did in the bathroom. I ain't your mama!

Lastly caregivers, watch your words. You don't have to believe what I do, but don't be a downer. Let the personality of the people you care for shine! Let go of your agenda and let them do what they want. Speak positive words as it refreshes them and gives them life. I have to share some stories of ridiculous caregivers, because we all need a laugh.

The Princess caregiver – This lady liked to wear high heels to work every day. I repeatedly told her that this was not practical because the way I transferred required me to put my feet against the sole of her shoe. She did not listen and continued to wear hooker boots to work. One glorious day, she came to work wearing the hooker boots AND a tiara. Because I enjoy entertainment as much as anybody, I sent her out back to pick up dog poop! Oh, if only I could have taken a picture of the Princess picking up turds in her tiara and heels!

The turkey crossing – I had a caregiver who was always very late, but at least she showed up, right? She usually wore pajamas to work and looked like she just rolled out of bed, but at least she showed up, right? One day she was over an hour late because turkeys were crossing the road. I did not doubt her because I lived on a mountain with lots of wildlife, but do you really think that wild turkeys would ignore something like a honk coming from a giant car rolling their way? What did she do, get out and hopscotch with them?

The clean-handed caregiver –I love clean hands, but I still have a hard time believing this really happened. After an outing, we were cleaning out the van. One caregiver gathered all the trash and handed it to the other caregiver who exclaimed that she couldn't take it because she had just washed her hands and they were clean. The fact that she was on the clock didn't seem to faze her!

The sleeping beauty – There once was a caregiver who was always so tired. She was so exhausted that she could not hold her head up. Her youth had apparently escaped her. During oral suction all caregivers stand, but not her. Not only was she seated, but this wand seemed to appear out of nowhere to suck my spit! I looked out of the corner of my eye to see that she was resting her poor little tuckered out head on the dresser next to my bed!! You for real?

CHAPTER EIGHT

BEWARE OF HOSPITALS AND FACILITIES

Not all hospitals and facilities are the same. Finally, I have found a hospital with wonderful staff that treat me like a human being! Their people are smiling and friendly every single time I visit. I have yet to have a bad experience. From the front desk to the lab to radiology to the ER to the ICU, they have great people! A big thank you to the people at McKee Hospital in Loveland, Colorado, for being different from the rest! This chapter is from my first book. I felt it was important to know this information for your survival.

I was not looking forward to writing this chapter, but you need to know what I didn't. I thought that the hospital was the safest place to be. Hospitals are not safe! I will list some things that happened to me without going into great detail. Keep in mind that I am no victim. God's eyes never close and He is my avenger.

When my husband went to pull up the car, two medical assistants got me out of bed and tried to make me walk to the wheelchair about five feet away. They didn't know I couldn't walk. When they pulled my arms to get me to stand, my head snapped back and stayed there. I was looking behind me with my head upside down. My ankles were rolled. They never asked me or even looked at my face. I could speak and the whole time I was yelling, "No, no, no! Stop!"

I was admitted to the hospital and my caregiver was told she had to leave (which is against the law when you are unable to speak for yourself). The doctor and team of nurses taped my arms down to two tables and tried to put in a urinary catheter. I don't need a catheter because I am continent and the idiots would have known that if they would have let my caregiver enter. They kept trying over and over to get the catheter inserted, which hurts! I now know that it is also against the law to restrain a patient.

During admitting I was given a wristband with the identity of an 87-year old man.

Once the nurse wouldn't stop touching me when I was telling her to stop. My caregiver had to grab her wrists to get her to stop.

I was given a bagging treatment based on another patient's x-ray, when my lungs were perfectly clear. The radiology department put my name on someone else's x-ray who happened to have a tube in his lungs.

The surgeon who did my tracheostomy took it upon herself to remove a large beauty mark off my neck that was nowhere near the incision site without my permission. It left a huge scar.

A nurse once tried to tell my caregivers to stop suctioning and to restrict it to once every four hours.

We were washing my hair in bed and had lowered the head of the bed so the basin would sit flat. When we were done, we raised the bed and because of the pooling in the lungs, it caused a secretion attack. These attacks lasted for hours. I once watched the sun come up with a caregiver and we were suctioning from 11pm to about 7am. This attack was different because it stopped abruptly. I felt something happening in my left lung. I told Megan to call the ambulance and we went to the hospital. The pulmonologist on call was a condescending pessimist who said it was not practical to suction as much as we did. He took an X-ray of my chest and because it was clear, tried to send me on my way. I insisted that there was something in my left lung and he finally said he would do a bronchoscopy. As he put the worm like thing into my lungs he said, there's nothing here. Then, lo and behold, he pulled out an 8-inch string of mucus that had many knots. Yeah, there's nothing here my ass!

After a routine trach change, a nurse anesthetist refused to let my caregivers care for me and slammed the ventilator onto my trach and used a thick foam pad around the trach instead of the usual thin gauze, causing me to bleed for hours. We suctioned blood out of my lungs for about three hours and then they told us we had to leave because they needed the room.

I was kicked out of the hospital after a two-week stay for refusing to take multiple laxatives per day because my poop was liquid. I was down to 75 pounds. I was labeled a refusing patient. I hung a sign on my door that read, "I refuse! I refuse to die. I refuse to give up. I refuse to let you take my joy!" The cause for this need for hospitalization was a home nurse who got me a prescription for a medication that was never indicated to be crushed for administration through a feeding tube. Also, she instructed me to increase the dose to a level that was an overdose. The medication destroyed the lining of my stomach. Never take medication without researching the drug first and know the correct dosage, administration and drug to drug interactions. I knew better, but I trusted her and the doctor who wrote the prescription.

*   *   *

Caregiver, you must be an advocate! Don't leave the person you're caring for alone. If all these things happened to me in just a few years, think about how common it must be that a patient's rights are violated. Before I found McKee, I cannot remember having a good experience at a hospital and the ones I have been to are considered great hospitals. Don't get me wrong, there have been some wonderful doctors and nurses, but the bad ones sort of ruin it for the good ones. It makes me angry enough to do something about it like go to law school and help create new laws to protect people who are in my situation. The following was taken from a brochure at my local hospital. Please request one if you are hospitalized or admitted to a facility and remember, you have the right to refuse anything!

Patient Rights (from MCR Hospital, Loveland, Colorado)

1. Receive quality care that is considerate and respectful of your dignity, personal values, beliefs and life philosophy.
2. Express your spiritual beliefs and cultural practices as long as they do not harm or interfere with your medical treatment or that of another patient.
3. Have your pain managed in the safest way possible.
4. Effective communication, regardless of language or other barriers.
5. Be involved in planning your care and to understand what is expected of you.
6. Refuse treatment as permitted by law and to be informed of the medical consequences of your decisions.
7. Be interviewed, examined, and treated in a safe setting that provides personal privacy.
8. Be free from all forms of abuse or harassment.

9.   A clear, concise explanation of your condition and proposed treatment.

10.   Know who is responsible for your care (physical and others) and their role here, including any relationship they may have to other health care providers or educational institutions.

11.   Be informed of hospitals rules and regulations that apply to your conduct.

12.   See your medical records within the guidelines established by law.

13.   Request a transfer to a different room if a suitable room for your care needs is available.

14.   Know in advance of any experimental, research or educational activities involved in your treatment. You can refuse to participate in any such activity.

15.   Be informed of your rights and responsibilities in a simple and easy to understand manner.

16.   Seek a medical ethics consultation if ethical issues arise.

17.   Create advance directives and have staff comply with them.

18.   Transfer to another facility, when medically permissible, if we are unable to meet your request or needs for care.

19. Have an authorized representative exercise your rights if you are unable to participate in your care or treatment decisions.

20. Receive a copy of your bill after you are discharged. You may request an explanation of charges, regardless of who is paying the bill.

21. Have your own doctor and a family member/ representative notified promptly of your admission to the hospital, as requested.

22. Be free from restraints of any form that are not medically necessary, including ones that are used as a means of coercion, discipline, convenience, or retaliation by staff.

23. Express any complaints and concerns, including those about patient care and safety.

24. Before starting care or treatment, you have the right to request information.
    - About the hospital's general billing procedures.
    - About usual and customary charges or estimated charges.

25. Designate visitors who will receive the same visitation privileges as your immediate family members, regardless of whether the visitors are legally related to you. The hospital will not deny

visitations privileges on the basis of race, color, national origin, religion, sex, sexual orientation, gender identity or disability.

CHAPTER NINE

IF YOU HAVE BEEN DIAGNOSED WITH ALS, THIS IS FOR YOU

If you have been diagnosed with a terminal disease, especially ALS, I cannot express how much I love you. I know what it's like. I know the deep pain and rejection you feel. People treat you differently. I see your posts on Facebook and I read your stories. You are each so precious. For those who have died and continue to die, I weep in my soul. There is a kinship I cannot explain. You are family. Because I love you, I tell you the truth. You do not have to accept this. It's just a diagnosis. I was also diagnosed with MS and PLS. If those diagnoses by world-renowned clinics were wrong, why can't the diagnosis of ALS end up being wrong? They conducted test after test to arrive at the diagnosis and they were still wrong! Doctors are so limited. Healing is real. Whether or not you believe in Jesus has nothing to do with it. Non-Christians get healed all the time because they believe. Having faith doesn't always mean having faith in God. Just because I think that being a Christian is the way to go doesn't mean that you have to agree to be healed. I want you healed. I also want you saved, but maybe that's too much for you right now. You say you don't know anyone who has been healed of ALS? I do! Tony Myers[9]! He is writing books about it. You can find him on Facebook.[10] You can listen to his healing testimony on YouTube.[11] Before you listen to it, you need to know that he was healed at home alone, because he believed!

You are not a person who HAS ALS, you're a person that was diagnosed with ALS. There is a difference. Sure, you have symptoms. Open your mind to the world of the unseen. Quantum physics, if you will. Everything we can see was made from the things that we cannot see. "Through faith we understand that the worlds were framed by the word of God, so that things which are seen were not made by the things which do appear". (Hebrews 11:3) Health can be made through things we cannot see. You're motor neurons are just waiting to be

---

[9] Tony Meyers' website: www.tonybelieves.com
[10] Tony Meyers' Facebook page:
https://www.facebook.com/tony.myers2
[11] Tony Meyers' Healing Testimony:
https://www.youtube.com/watch?v=xkc750AF2U4

reactivated. They are listening to your words. They are activated by faith.

You are blessed and cannot be cursed unless you don't know it and curse yourself. "Christ hath redeemed us from the curse of the law becoming a curse for us, for it is written, cursed is anyone who hangeth on a tree, that the blessings of Abraham might come upon the gentiles through Christ." (Galatians 3:13)

The Curse of the Law

What is the curse that you have already been redeemed from? ALS and so much more! For the full curse that you have been redeemed from, check out Deuteronomy 28:15-68. Notice it says, 'prolonged sicknesses.' That's us! It also says that every sickness and every plague is included in the curse and we have been redeemed from them all! Here's just a small portion of the physical curses that you have been redeemed from (and there are financial curses too!):

"If you do not carefully observe all the words of this law that are written in this book, that you may fear this glorious and awesome name, THE LORD YOUR GOD, then the LORD will bring upon you and your descendants extraordinary plagues—great and prolonged plagues—and serious and **prolonged sicknesses**. Moreover He will bring back on you all the diseases of Egypt, of which you were afraid, and they shall cling to you. Also **every sickness and every plague**, which *is* not written in this Book of the Law, will the LORD bring upon you until you are destroyed. You shall be left few in number, whereas you were as the stars of heaven in multitude, because you would not obey the voice of the LORD your God. And it shall be, *that* just as the LORD rejoiced over you to do you good and multiply you, so the LORD will rejoice over you to destroy you and bring you to nothing; and you shall be plucked from off the land which you go to possess." (Deuteronomy 28:58-63)

The Blessings

Below is how you are blessed. The thing that most people don't understand is that Jesus obeyed the voice of the Lord and every commandment on YOUR behalf! When people read the part about obeying the commandments, they know they can't and forget the whole thing. We never have been able to obey and fulfil the law. That's why Jesus obeyed for you! This is why

Christian's are nuts about Jesus. I explain this because I didn't understand this for a long time. Jesus made it possible for us to be qualified for the blessings and redeemed from the curse. We didn't have to do squat!

All we have to do is believe!

"Now it shall come to pass, if you diligently obey the voice of the LORD your God, to observe carefully all His commandments which I command you today, that the LORD your God will set you high above all nations of the earth. And all these blessings shall come upon you and overtake you, because you obey the voice of the LORD your God:

"Blessed *shall* you *be* in the city, and blessed *shall* you *be* in the country. Blessed *shall be* the fruit of your body, the produce of your ground and the increase of your herds, the increase of your cattle and the offspring of your flocks. Blessed *shall be* your basket and your kneading bowl. Blessed *shall* you *be* when you come in, and blessed *shall* you *be* when you go out. The LORD will cause your enemies who rise against you to be defeated before your face; they shall come out against you one way and flee before you seven ways.

The LORD will command the blessing on you in your storehouses and in all to which you set your hand, and He will bless you in the land which the LORD your God is giving you. The LORD will establish you as a holy people to Himself, just as He has sworn to you, if you keep the commandments of the LORD your God and walk in His ways. Then all peoples of the earth shall see that you are called by the name of the LORD, and they shall be afraid of you. And the LORD will grant you plenty of goods, in the fruit of your body, in the increase of your livestock, and in the produce of your ground, in the land of which the LORD swore to your fathers to give you. The LORD will open to you His good treasure, the heavens, to give the rain to your land in its season, and to bless all the work of your hand. You shall lend to many nations, but you shall not borrow. And the LORD will make you the head and not the tail; you shall be above only, and not be beneath, if you heed the commandments of the LORD your God, which I command you today, and are careful to observe *them*. So you shall not turn aside from any of the words which I command you this day, *to* the right or the left, to go after other gods to serve them." (Deuteronomy 28:1-14)

This is good news. We have already been blessed with everything mentioned above. We will not experience it unless we agree with it and align our words and actions with it. Are you always tired of being below circumstances and not above? Do you say things like, under the circumstances, I am okay. Get out from under your circumstances! Act and speak like you're above your circumstances and you WILL be!

CHAPTER *TEN*

FAITH AND FAST FOOD

Before I wrote this chapter, I had to solidify what it is that I believe. Faith evolves and some things that you used to believe, change. I study and will listen to the same audiobooks over and over. Free audiobooks on YouTube are the best! I listen to them all night long and then when I wake up, I learn something and go back to sleep. I have often thought that I am spiritually slow. I would listen to super Christians say, 'all you have to do is believe and receive!' While that is true, I didn't get it. Religious people have made it difficult for people to receive. They create so many requirements and rules to be able to receive. I don't think that God can be painted into a box so easily. I have chosen to be a Christian because I believe it is the right thing, but being a Christian asks you to believe in things that are pretty crazy. God is three-in-one? God in person form was born to a virgin? And then died and raised from the dead by the Holy Spirit? No wonder people think Christians are nuts!

Christians will not like me for this, but you don't have to believe in God to be healed. People of many different religions are healed simply because of belief! God has made our brains with the absolutely amazing ability to believe. As I began studying things like the law of attraction, I felt like I was cheating on God. There are many Law of Attraction teachers that are not Christian. They do not give the credit to God and give all the glory to the universe, which rubs me the wrong way. I have come to the conclusion that God is the one behind everything good and He designed us this way. If they want to talk about it being the universe instead of God, they are the ones who are missing out.

It is a big relief to know that you don't need to be Christian to believe and have circumstances change in your life. It releases people from the requirements. I don't think preachers realize how they frame healing sometimes. They say, all you have to do is believe... and then they add ten things you have to do. I love God and I am so thankful I know Him. I just think that many preachers miss the point. Many people are healed at the grotto in Lourdes, France. It is not because the grotto or the water is special. It's because people expect to be healed and believe! It helps me to know that nobody in the Bible who was healed was a Christian. If all these heathens got healed, why not us heathens? We are just as qualified as anyone else.

Let's proceed, heathens. It is in the believing, whether it's that Jesus has already healed you (because He has) or you can have your subconscious healing you. Take it anyway it comes! I can already hear Christians getting upset with me. Okay, Jesus is my Lord and Savior, so back down. I want to help people have hope and get well. I have wasted years under preaching that disqualified me. You cannot deny the healings that take place outside of Christianity. I want to lead people to the Lord just like you do, but we are chasing them away by our approach. The truth is that we can be healed by believing we are healed! The truth is also that healing is included in salvation and I will get to that.

First let's talk about learning how the mind works. This is so fascinating! God rocks! He made it so that when we think about good things, we get more good things and when we focus on the bad, we get more bad. This is the law of attraction. This is something I understand and can do! Energy flows where focus goes. Several times a day I close my eyes and think: I am well, well-being is surrounding every cell of my body. Or, I am healthy, I am strong and I am able to do everything I need and want to do with my body. "Call those things that be not as if they were." (Romans 4:17) The full scripture is even more awesome. "As it is written, I have made you a father of many nations, in the presence of God in whom he believed, who gives life to the dead and calls into existence the things that do not yet exist." God called Abraham a father of many nations before he had children and he calls each and every one of us healed today. As I say that I am well, I am calling into existence a thing that does not yet exist! This is powerful and exciting and it's something I can do about my situation instead of griping.

For how the subconscious works, I am going to refer you to some awesome audiobooks because I am still learning myself. I will tell you that this information on how the mind works will blow you away. So often we attract the things we fear the most. If instead, we just focused on the good, our worst fears never would have happened. What we didn't know has been hurting us. If you only study two books, study these two (and they are free on YouTube):

The Secret by Rhonda Byrne (different than the documentary below)

The Magic of Believing by Claude Bristol

These books will change your life if you study them. They have certainly changed mine. Listen to them continuously all throughout the year. I also recommend watching the documentary 'The Secret' on Netflix about one hundred times. In the documentary, there is a man who was in a plane crash and his body was destroyed. He was on a ventilator and all he could do was blink his eyes. Sound familiar? I love his story and you will have to watch it! Start using your faith on symptoms. Make faith a habit. Recently, I used my faith and had wonderful results. I bit the head off of my electric toothbrush because I am vicious! Uhh, I bit it off because of a hyper reflex combined with spasticity. I severed the steel pen that attached the head. It left my mouth with deep cuts inside and out, and I got a fat lip I didn't even have to pay for! After five days of putting essential oils in my mouth and on my lips, I thought, this is stupid-it's gone! I believed it with my heart and by the next day it was healed. I didn't even check it because the pain was gone. Pretty cool, huh? I totally felt it in my heart. I was mad about the stupid thing and tired of people putting hands in my mouth. Now If I can just get that mad about the rest of my body, I will come visit you until you're healed!

I will work for food. I am a fat girl on the inside. I dream about lying on the floor at Taco Bell and opening my mouth while someone turns the nacho cheese valve. I have visions of going through the drive-thru in my mini cooper that I will have again, ordering two Taco Supremes and about a dozen bean burritos (old habits die hard - it's the cheapest thing on the menu) parking where nobody can see me and scarfing violently until my pants don't fit! If you have ever tasted Taco Bell's sour cream, you understand that it's magical. It is full fat and I am guessing straight from Mexico because it's hard to find full fat sour cream in the States, I've looked. Yes! I can't wait! Oh I know, you thought I was so polished and refined. Hate to burst your bubble! After not eating for six years by mouth, I am an animal!

Okay, I have to tell you about my other vision just in case you work at Wendy's and hear about it. I don't know why I am dining inside on this particular day, maybe the line is too long at the drive-thru or something. Clearly I value wrapping my neglected taste buds around some deliciousness over protecting my dignity. I order one of everything pretty much so the employees are already looking at me funny because I am alone. Burgers with bacon, chili, a loaded baked potato, fries with a hundred of those little ketchup cups you have to pump, a fried chicken sandwich, and a fish sandwich extra tartar extra pickle (I have researched this and they hold the top ranking for a fish sandwich among all fast food restaurants, sorry Filet-o-fish you blow). As I take the first bite, tears start streaming down my face and with burgers in hands, I raise my hands praising God for this food. It's so delicious! I have never tasted anything so good in all my life! The bacon? Tears. The chili with extra cheese? Tears. I dip the potato into the chili and sink my teeth in. Thank you God! Funny, I never dream about salad.

I must move on because I am salivating and need sukilicious (oral suction) in a big way! This is what it's about folks. Finding the things that excite you and meditating on them until you salivate or feel it in your body. I literally look up menus and have had caregivers read me menus in a very slow seductive voice. I am surprised that my cholesterol is not through the roof it feels so real. I don't watch much TV, but I love 'Somebody Feed Phil' and 'I'll Have What Phil's Having' on Netflix. I will go to the Cordon Blue in Paris and become a chef in Jesus' name. Then I can come back and cook for you hungry bastards.

Let's get serious. God loves you so much and wants you healed anyway it comes. He also wants a relationship with you. When you do get healed, God and I hope you see that it is from Him and cuddle up! He sent Jesus to reconcile us with God because we are screw ups. When Jesus went to the cross to be crucified, he was beaten so we could be healed. That was two thousand years ago. Why would he do that? Love. You were healed. You've already got it. Thank him for it, talk like it, think like it, act like it. Believe!

ADDITIONAL RESOURCES:

https://www.awmi.net/video/healing/

https://www.awmi.net/audio/audio-
teachings/#/awm_1033a_blessed.mp3

Billy Burke:
https://www.youtube.com/watch?v=Av0ArUM65LI&t=47s

It is a little known fact that after Jesus gave the
commandment to love one another, he said "every church
must have a black choir to invigorate thy people." Here's a
lady whose spirit we need to catch!
https://www.youtube.com/watch?v=Pk_1ZE7Rwcg

This is beautiful, powerful and puts things in perspective:
https://www.youtube.com/watch?v=d3jgPsGQSdQ

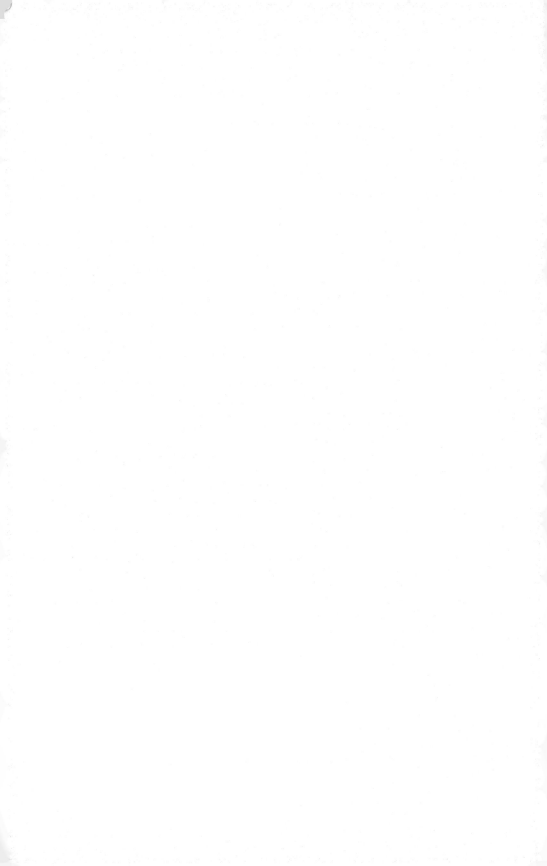

Printed in Great Britain
by Amazon

83989852R00089